Born Submissive

I Was Raised in a BDSM Household

by
Deanna Hankel

Moons Grove Press
British Columbia, Canada

Born Submissive: I Was Raised in a BDSM Household

Copyright ©2022 by Deanna Hankel
ISBN-13 978-1-77143-511-6
First Edition

Library and Archives Canada Cataloguing in Publication
Title: Born submissive : I was raised in a BDSM household /
by Deanna Hankel.
Names: Hankel, Deanna, 1967- author.
Identifiers: Canadiana (print) 20220138508 | Canadiana (ebook) 20220138680
| ISBN 9781771435116 (softcover) | ISBN 9781771435123 (PDF)
Subjects: LCSH: Hankel, Deanna. | LCSH: Sexual dominance and submission.
| LCSH: Bondage (Sexual behavior) | LCSH: Sadomasochism.
| LCSH: Sadomasochists—Biography. | LCGFT: Autobiographies.
Classification: LCC HQ79 .H36 2022 | DDC 306.77/5092—dc23

Artwork credit: Front and back cover artwork © Deanna Hankel

Moons Grove Press is an imprint
of CCB Publishing: www.ccbpublishing.com

Moons Grove Press
British Columbia, Canada
www.moonsgrovepress.com

To my Dominant,
who showed me what I already knew,
that I was born submissive

Contents

Introduction vii

PART I

Chapter 1   D/s: Identity or Activity? 1

Chapter 2   What Kind of D/s Relationship
             Do You Want? 5

Chapter 3   Consent (Or Lack of Consent) 11

Chapter 4   Training 19

Chapter 5   Conditioning 27

Chapter 6   The History of BDSM 33

PART II

Chapter 7   Punishment 39

Chapter 8   Journaling 45

Chapter 9   Mind Games 49

Chapter 10   Bondage & Humiliation 53

Chapter 11   Devaluation 57

Chapter 12   Taskmaster 63

PART III

Chapter 13   BDSM Toys 69

Chapter 14   Taskmaster II (The Sadist Boss) 75

Chapter 15   Taskmaster III (The Dominant Boss) 79

Chapter 16   Domestic Service 83

Chapter 17   Sexting 89

Chapter 18   Finding the Right Dominant 97

Reader Bonus –
    A teaser of Deanna Hankel's memoir
    Trapped in the 70s: Behind A Sadist's Door 103

References 107

INTRODUCTION

I was born to a submissive mother and a Dominant father and am quite happy to be a submissive, which is a good thing because I also don't know any other way to be. As you may know, BDSM isn't always about sex. Sometimes it's only about power. Therefore, it's important to understand that it's possible to grow up in a BDSM household without ever having participated in BDSM sex. I believe that the power exchange will still permeate the air the way an electric current flows when electrons move through a conductor. I also believe it's extremely important to know your own strengths and weaknesses in order to know who you are, as well as your backstory, so here's a bit of mine.

My father engaged in heavy domination with males, perhaps even as far back as before my parents' marriage. This provocative fact was not revealed until after their divorce in the 1970s. My mother, a highly obedient submissive, later remarried a bonafide sadist, which gives yet another perspective on the world of BDSM. She and my stepfather had a Master/slave relationship with no boundaries. She gave up all of her rights and lived a pretty frightening and uncomfortable life, in my opinion. I, however, chose a D/s relationship as an adult, which I find highly fulfilling.

The purpose of this book is to make you *feel* like you've lived in both a Master/slave and a D/s household. You'll be able to see through my eyes what it's like to be both a slave and a submissive. I'll take you through the halls of a sadist's house, where a Doberman Pinscher stood guard and awaited his Master's training command: *Kill*. You'll also roam the halls of a highly particular Dominant's house and experience what it's like to have D/s sex on what he refers to as "my wall." You'll then be able to make an informed choice about the type of BDSM relationship you want.

BDSM stands for bondage and discipline, dominance and submission, and sadism and masochism. But what exactly is a submissive? You might be aware of the power exchange that takes place between a Dominant and a submissive, where the latter gives all of her power up to her Dominant after some boundaries have been set. If so, then hopefully, you are also aware that the submissive may take back any or all of that power at any time. You may also be aware of the arrangement between Master and slave, where the slave gives up all of her power to her Master along with all of her property without having set any boundaries. In that case, I hope once again you are aware that the slave may take back any or all of that power at any time. The power is always yours to exchange.

By the way, as a daughter of a bisexual male from the leather culture, I am fully aware that Dominants, submissives, Masters, and slaves can be either male or female and that males may even corner the market on the BDSM world. This book, however, is based on my life experience as a submissive, so it's told from the female submissive's point of view. I hope that no males will be offended any more than I am offended because some can walk in heels better than I can.

Born Submissive

Part I

ℰ Chapter 1 ℭ

D/s: Identity or Activity?

L et's get right down to it, shall we? Is D/s about who you are or an activity in which you wish to engage? You'll want to narrow this down the same way a writer will want to narrow down the tone so he'll have a focused story. So let's start with your character. First of all, you'll want to determine whether you're a submissive or a slave. And what exactly is a slave, you ask? A slave only wants to serve completely and—dare I say—blindly? She simply wants to please her Master solely for the privilege of continuing to serve so that she feels complete. Not a thought does she give to her own personal needs other than food and shelter. Anything else is granted by the grace of her Master at his whim. Does this sound like you, or does it sound a bit too extreme for your tastes?

I, myself, prefer being a submissive to being a slave. Although I may have been a slave in my past life somewhere back in the Middle Ages, it's not who I am. I'm a submissive because I have submitted to my Dominant. I also obey him and accept the consequences for disobedience, which leave me breathless and tingly each and every time. One reason is that the consequences come with both the promise (or anticipation) and delivery (or execution) of his full attention and ownership of me. It thrills me to my core each time he calls me his "owned bitch" and sends me to my knees. It also keeps me crawling back for more.

If you have to ask yourself whether you're inherently Dominant or submissive, you're probably part of the large percentage who are both. Some believe that 10% are true Dominants, and 10% are true submissives. But what about those whose occupation defies their core personality? Some Dominants tire of cracking the whip all day and find themselves wanting to hand it over at night. They can be hard to spot, so it's best not to assume someone fits into one role or another. This does not describe a "switch," which is someone who enjoys switching from a Dominant to a submissive role. So are they a closet Dominant in the same way that a gay person might be a closet homosexual?

This is where it gets interesting (not that the entire world of BDSM isn't interesting). It's widely accepted that the human race is sexual and that those of us in the gay community who are not "out and proud" are said to be "in the closet." So what about BDSM, which is not largely accepted? Aren't most Dominants already "in the closet" for this very reason? So then, are the Dominants who want to hand over the whip in the bedroom included in the 10% of those who are true Dominants, or are they in a separate category of "closet, closet Dominants?" My point is that labels are probably a silly and overly simplistic way of defining people, who have approximately 100 billion brain cells that make up their unique personality. Labels are more like adjectives that one uses to describe something, and we all know there's always more than one adjective from which to choose. Therefore, labels are more of a form of reference.

So when I use the label "true Dominant," it by no means reflects my thoughts about the validity or purity of the personality. On the contrary, it's simply my way of explaining the personality to which I'm referring at the time. Remember, I'm a submissive, and as a submissive, I genuinely believe that it's the man who makes the man, not the label. Having said that, I'm now going to describe what I believe to be a "true Dominant." This individual doesn't know any other way to be and would find it against his nature to assume the role of a submissive in any arena. I believe this is also true of a true submissive, who would be extremely uncomfortable taking on a Dominant role. If you can't relate to either of these feelings, then chances are you're probably in the large percentage outside of these two, and I don't dare speculate about the "true number."

If you're simply open to trying BDSM as a way to spice up your sex life, that's fine as long as you and your partner are both on the same page and one of you isn't pressuring the other into trying to be something they're not. On the other hand, if one of you doesn't feel they can live without BDSM and the other finds it isn't for them, you might have a problem. It's vitally important for any relationship that the partners share the same values and vision. You should also understand what you're getting into and whether or not it's for you. And if you're wondering whether you're a bedroom submissive or lifestyle submissive, here are some questions you might want to consider:

Do you find yourself drawn to confident, assertive men? Are you able to immediately spot them in a crowd? Do they make you giddy and cause your hand to fly up to your throat? Many true submissives have an inherent ability to spot them. They can quickly pick out the alpha male in a room or even in a photograph. The way a man walks and carries himself says a lot about what's in his head. If you find poor posture to be a complete turnoff, you might just be a submissive.

Does it make you happy to provide service to someone you love? Do you long to serve and give of yourself without any thought of receiving in return? Performing service can be very fulfilling, but do you also find yourself sacrificing your own comfort for others? Have you ever found yourself taken advantage of because of your eagerness to serve? If so, then you might be a submissive.

Do you go out of your way to avoid confrontation at all costs? Does the thought bring you extreme anxiety and discomfort, perhaps to the point of nausea? There are generally two types of people when it comes to dealing with confrontation: those who seek it out and enjoy it and those who run from it. If you're the latter, you might be a submissive.

Does the idea of having to make crucial decisions on your own bring you distress? Are you afraid the choice you make might somehow interfere with your relationship? Perhaps that career move might detract from your duties at home. For each of us, there are hundreds of decisions that we must make daily. Do you often find yourself asking your partner for advice or guidance about them? If so, you might be a submissive.

So now what?

❧ Chapter 2 ❧

What Kind of D/s Relationship Do You Want?

Are you ready for a lifestyle D/s relationship where your Dominant has control of you both inside and outside of the bedroom? Have you seriously considered the prospect of having to request permission or report all self-pleasuring sessions to him? Are you prepared for serving and service to become your primary purpose in life? Are you willing to give up your right to personal choice? How would you feel about being told by your Dominant that your trip to the market should take no more than forty-five minutes? Are you willing to accept the prospect of correction being administered by your Dominant should the trip have taken longer than his projected time? Perhaps you remembered some clothes that needed picking up from the drycleaners. Will your Dominant find this to be a willful display of independence? Will you be punished for such insubordination?

So, what are the benefits of having a D/s relationship? Believe me, there are more than I can count. For example, I often feel the overwhelming need to be pulled by the hair, pushed onto the floor, and firmly ordered around by my Dominant. I can even hear his voice in my head during the day when he's not around, that voice which says, "I'm all man, and I'm taking you." I crave him putting me in my place and letting me know where I belong: at his feet. I need my Dominant's hand on my throat, stifling my breath while the other is spanking my ass until it's red. But for me to submit to him, I had to trust him with not only my body but my mind. Only then could I truly surrender.

So why do you want a D/s relationship? Is your purpose to achieve a relationship that's free of a power struggle? Do you want a Dominant who puts as much effort into the relationship as you do? If so, you should first take a look at yourself. Do you know who you are? Have you learned from your past mistakes? Do you admit when you're wrong? Are you able to effectively communicate your needs and issues?

The method by which we communicate should be tailored to suit the person with whom we're communicating. After all, you wouldn't speak to a child the same way you'd speak to an adult. So how about your Dominant? Does he think in visual terms? If so, would watching a film about a particular issue help him relate to the situation? Does he think in spatial terms? If so, would drawing a diagram be helpful to him?

And what type of lifestyle do you want? Are you looking for private parties with your Dominant on his wall, or are you looking to bounce off walls at the local BDSM dungeon? Are you able to express your kinky fantasies to your Dominant without fear that he'll think less of you? Are you willing to accommodate his kinky desires even if they make you nervous?

And how important is it to you that your Dominant be enlightened? Would it be enough that he's open to exploring consciousness with you? What about shared values? It might be a good idea to sit down with him and discuss each other's values. This will also help you both discover each other's core beliefs. The more you know about yourself and your Dominant, the better you'll be able to work together as one.

It's also critical to work through each other's personal values, hopes, dreams, wants, needs, and fears. And what does domination mean to each of you? Perhaps domination to one of you means ordering for the other at dinner, but to the other, it means ordering oral sex beneath the table during a conference call with their boss.

How about your image? Are you obsessed with it? Do you hide behind your mask? You should ask yourself what you think people are saying behind your back at work. If the answer describes the image you're projecting rather than the real you, you'll want to do some work on yourself before getting into a new relationship.

Here are some traits a submissive might want to seek out in a potential Dominant: Someone who's emotionally and physically strong; Someone who's responsible; Someone who wants to grow both emotionally and spiritually; Someone who possesses enough knowledge and life experience to serve as a mentor; Someone who's able to correct and discipline the submissive, but does so in a safe environment; Someone who communicates effectively; Someone who's honest; Someone who'll appreciate you.

Here are some traits a Dominant might seek out in a potential submissive: Someone who's experienced in the art of service; Someone who has high ethics and morals; Someone who's positive; Someone who's nurturing and empathetic; Someone who's a quick learner; Someone who can adapt to new situations; Someone who's able to act during situations rather than react due to issues from their past; Someone who's flexible enough to be able to adapt to the tastes of the Dominant over their own; Someone who's adventurous.

What kind of service skills do you have to offer? Some appropriate skills for a submissive might include speaking well, dressing well, being well-read, knowing art, music, dance, and secretarial skills. What about personal habits such as disorganization? Do you know where everything is in your home? Is everything in its place or strewn about the house? For example, in my household, items are appropriately categorized into labeled bins. It's clear where to find any item related to electronics, tools, office supplies, etc. As for the bathroom, items are not cluttering up the counter; they are laid out on a tray that can be easily lifted for cleaning.

However, my Dominant sometimes finds it irritating when I do things such as close up a box of pie that he was planning to revisit or immediately put away his pen. After the first year with someone, you should know whether you would be able to live with the other person's personal habits. For example, my ex-husband always arose at 5 am so that he could read *Investor's Business Daily* before the stock market opened. This meant that not only was he in bed by 10 pm, but the schedule also included weekends because he could no longer sleep past 5 am. His personal schedule never actually presented a problem for me until he purchased a piece of home gym equipment, which he placed inside the bedroom suite for 5 am workouts.

What kinds of personal habits annoy you? How about a Dominant who spends all of his extra time and cash fixing up old cars? What about one who travels on business for two-thirds of the year? What about a Dominant who's only formal wear consists of a tuxedo printed on a t-shirt? You might want to think about the long-term effects that habits like these could have on your relationship. Don't rush the period when the two of you are getting to know each other.

So, what kinds of people make good D/s partners? You might think that both need to be serious adventure-seekers, but that might lead to them being risk-takers. This is why it's important to have well-defined boundaries. When well-defined boundaries have been established, then play will be enjoyed within a safe environment. It's always better to have one person who keeps the other in check rather than two people who want to live on the edge.

So, what kind of Dominant attracts you? How would you feel about a man who didn't stand up for himself in a business situation? What about a man who didn't stand up for you against another man in a bar? How about a man with a high voice? What image do you project that would attract the type of man that you seek? Does your online dating profile portray you in all camouflage, holding a rifle, and saying that you would make a good hunting buddy, or are there some dresses in your closet that would show your feminine side?

Would the two of you make a good couple? When you're in a relationship, do you tend to overlook some issues that the two of you are having because you want things to work? Perhaps you wish he wasn't so messy, and perhaps he wishes you didn't repeat yourself so often. These little things can be negotiated, but sexual incompatibility cannot. If one person likes to have sex once a week and the other prefers sex twice a day, that could be a problem. If one person cannot satisfy the other person sexually, that could also be a problem. This is because most people would prefer not to say anything than hurt the other person's feelings or ego. Over time, this can lead to problems.

For those of us in a D/s relationship, it gets even more complicated. What if you need to be hog-tied to get into a scene, but your Dominant needs to see you lowered onto his cock by a rope? And make sure you know what turns you on because, for those of us in the BDSM world, it may take that special person who's willing to pull out our brand of kink.

Now it's time to decide how much effort you're willing to put into the relationship. It takes a lot of work for two people to become a couple. There's obedience and protocols to be learned by the submissive and management skills to be learned or honed by the Dominant. He may already be a manager for his occupation or may want to consider reading some books about leadership. Some of the skills include executing commands, good listening skills, patience, humility, and emotional intelligence. Looking for a Dominant who already has some management experience will be the preferred route.

ᘒ Chapter 3 ᘓ

Consent
(Or Lack of Consent)

I'd like you to imagine a hypothetical example of standing in the nude looking at a man who's also in the nude because you are nudists, he says. Suppose you're in South Florida, where it rarely gets cold, but you're being told to ask permission of this man to wear clothes whenever it does get cold. And this man may say no. He has not told you to address him as Master, nor has he told you to call him Sir. All you know is that his rules are yours to follow. He decides what you will eat and when and where you will eat it. He also decides that you will not be given a key to his house, and he decides that you will visit a nudist colony whenever he pleases. You have no idea of the concept of consenting to submit to someone else's will. All you know is that you have been told to follow this man's rules. Your friends do not walk around in the nude at home, nor do any of your extended relatives. But then you're made to go to a nudist colony, and you see that some people do. So now what? What is normal?

According to the dictionary, normal is what's usual, typical, or expected, and abnormal deviates from what's normal or usual in an undesirable or worrying way. It's funny to think that what some would find undesirable others might find to be quite desirable. Personally, as a writer, I feel it's our differences that make us interesting. There are many walks of life out there, and not all do what's usual, typical, or expected. For example, some enjoy the painful pleasure of having their hair pulled during sex. I happen to be one of them. But what exactly about this is pleasurable? Could it be the erotic construction of power exchange that has taken place between two consenting individuals when a submissive has willingly and voluntarily relinquished control to her Dominant?

Now I'd like you to imagine another hypothetical example where a stranger has pulled your hair on the street. They've snuck up behind you, grabbed hold of your locks, and yanked. Do you still think you'd find it pleasurable? No? Why? Because the consent is missing. Once the power exchange is gone, the erotic imagination is no longer involved, and now all that's left is the pain. We don't have the right to inflict pain on other people without their consent—that's referred to as assault. We also shouldn't devalue or humiliate people during sex without their consent and without making sure they know why we're doing it because, without the involvement of their erotic imagination, it's just emotional pain. It's like asking them to play a game but refusing to tell them the rules or, worse, not even letting them in on the fact that a game is being played at all. That just makes you a person who doesn't care whether your partner enjoys the pain. Instead, you just enjoy being cruel.

What if you haven't given your consent to be completely conditioned to obey someone else's will and are not even aware that there's such a thing as BDSM? For example, what if the nightly inspections of the sink to make sure you've scrubbed it well enough with scouring powder and the little notes on some food in the fridge telling you not to eat it are presented as normal? But where are the rewards from your Dominant? And where's the reward of feeling like a good submissive? Not a very fair game without consent being asked and given, is it?

There was a point in the relationship with my current Dominant when he asked me if I wanted to submit to him. We had been dating for some time and had had sex a couple of times, during which he had explained three of his personal rules to me. For example, he had told me that he would be the one directing all of the activity and that there were only two things he wanted to hear out of me when we were in bed: 1) yes, Sir, and 2) thank you, Sir. He also told me that that was how I was to address him whenever we were in private. The requests were all new to me; however, they felt perfectly natural and acceptable. So did the request to submit to him. Then he asked me *why* I wanted to submit to him.

Some submissives wish to submit to their Dominant because it turns them on to give him what he wants. Others are turned on by the primal power dynamic between a man and a woman. My reason, however, came to me immediately and ran extremely deep for me. It was also both a confession and a relief. I answered, "Because I don't know any other way to be." My Dominant, of course, then wanted to know why. "Because I've always been this way," I admitted, which only led to more questions than answers for him. Had I engaged in BDSM before with someone else? Not to my knowledge, I told him. Then had someone been telling me what to do? Yes, everyone, I'd told him. That's when he explained to me that it wasn't the same thing. "Well, it feels the same," I told him, which only caused him to become even more adamant about the fact that it wasn't.

"There has to be consent," he said. A good Dominant should ask you, his prospective submissive, if you want to submit to him well before any BDSM takes place. This is a big decision, and you need to be given time to make it. You may also need to be educated about the practices of BDSM. It's both your responsibility and the Dominant's responsibility to make sure you understand all that's involved. There should be no surprises. A person cannot agree to something to which they don't know they're agreeing.

For example, what about that prod-style electric shock device to correct bad behavior that you had no idea about? Or that bondage rack with weights and clamps? Clear boundaries need to be set about what kind of play will be allowed. There may be soft boundaries that are open to "pushing" by the Dominant, and there may be hard boundaries that are completely off-limits, such as water sports, where urinating and defecating are involved. There are plenty of BDSM lists on the Internet. Take a look at a few of them and decide what is and what is not acceptable to you.

You'll also want to make sure that you don't fall prey to sub-frenzy, which is a common mistake of new submissives. It's natural to want to be the best submissive possible and have no limits, but this is bound to cause you some pain. For example, don't agree to have a threesome with your Dominant because you think it will please him only to find yourself hurt in the process. Remember, the power exchange is for both of your enjoyment, not just your Dominant's.

You also want to make sure to be very specific when you set your boundaries. This is why some Dominants and submissives create and sign a contract. You can find many sample BDSM contracts online, but you should make sure to tailor it to your specific needs.

Not all Dominants and submissives use written contracts. Some even go as far as having a fancy binder with a lock and key. For others, an oral contract is sufficient. Of course, the more detailed and lengthy the list of limits, the more there is to remember. Some also wish to have their rituals written into the contract, as well. Rituals can help Dominants and submissives get back into their roles when everyday life pulls them in another direction. For example, the submissive may assume a slave position with her wrists crossed behind her back whenever her Dominant summons her. She may also assume a slave kneeling position upon her Dominant's command. Words may be exchanged during the ritual, as well.

The Dominant may ask, "Why are you my submissive?" and the submissive may respond, "Because I gave you all of my power, Sir."

This is where my conditioning comes in for me. I don't need any reminders to help me remember my place. I never forget. Years of living with the ever-present undercurrent of a BDSM household have left me in an ever-servicing state. I wouldn't think of questioning my Dominant. It simply wouldn't happen. I'm also quieter than a lot of people. When you leave out the arguing, the demanding, the complaining, and many of the opinions, there isn't nearly as much left to say. But I do express myself with my writing, and I suggest you do the same. There will be more on the subject of writing in the chapter on journaling.

Because I'm a writer, I love the differences in people and believe that our personalities make us suited for different types of relationships. I don't believe that everyone should be a submissive, nor do I believe that everyone should be a Dominant. That's what makes us interesting. I don't have all the answers, and I wasn't given a choice about who I am. I'm a submissive.

Having said that, I do feel that submitting to my Dominant keeps the household and our relationship running smoothly and makes for a conflict-free environment, the latter of which is critical to me. As a natural submissive, I tend to avoid conflict at all costs; however, I have gone through great pains to face my fears through writing. My process has usually been to draft several versions of a letter to my Dominant, give him the letter to read, and then get up the nerve to actually speak to him about the issue. The process took up the better part of our relationship's first year, and I'm happy to say that I'm now able to voice my concerns to him without always writing a letter. There's no more freezing up in front of him to the point where he suggests we put off the discussion for a couple of days or perhaps a week, hoping that it will just go away. It never does, so it's better to learn how to face conflict. I've learned this the hard way.

However, there's something to be said about having clearly defined roles. We see this work at the office with the employer/employee relationship, so why shouldn't the same process be implemented at home? Of course, there are good bosses and bad bosses. It's crucial to choose a good boss or Dominant who's just as interested in meeting your needs as you are in meeting his. And a good boss or Dominant should choose a good employee who's not lazy. I'm a big believer in the law of inertia, which states that an object at rest stays at rest, and an object in motion stays in motion. This law applies to all of us as humans, as well. Have you ever noticed that the more you neglect a duty because you simply don't feel like doing it, the less you will feel like doing it in the future? Then the next thing you know, there's a pile of dishes in the sink, and you and your partner haven't had sex in three weeks. Laziness has no place in a D/s relationship.

But how does it feel to be a submissive, you ask? Ah, that's the question. Is it all just about maintaining order in my life and house and avoiding conflict? No, it's not, although those are both big ones for me. I have to say that the best part about being a submissive for me is the connection it allows me to have with my Dominant. The clearly defined roles of our D/s relationship bring us so closely together that we truly feel like two halves of a whole. We know each other's core needs and desires and want to meet them. How many times have you heard the expression, "They just don't understand me?" That phrase should never be heard in a D/s relationship. The purpose of the journaling phase is to allow your Dominant to get into your head and explore both your triggers and desires. He may, in turn, decide to share his journaling with you, but even if he doesn't, you'll be able to see inside his head, as well, simply by the way he responds to your triggers and desires.

For example, does your Dominant respect your triggers and stop the scene to administer aftercare? This is the time you and your Dominant take after sex to recover and care for each other's physical and emotional needs. And how about your fantasies? Is your Dominant open to indulging in them with you? Journaling can be a very eye-opening experience for both of you.

ᐲ Chapter 4 ᐳ

Training

The D/s relationship may be summed up with this initial order by the Dominant to his sub: You will do exactly as instructed, and I will do exactly as I please. Most BDSM books have a section on training a submissive or "sub" to do exactly as her Dominant pleases. Still, I've decided to break the subject up into two chapters, Training and Conditioning. I've done this because I feel that training is more about the Dominant—learning his likes and dislikes—and that conditioning is more about the sub. The level of expertise that a Dominant will expect from his sub will vary. Some will want their sub to take classes in subjects such as ballroom dancing and flower arranging. They may even want to pick out their sub's clothes for them each day. Some are only particular about their food and will be very specific about the way they want everything to be cooked. And some are only interested in their sub's expertise in the bedroom, as the sole purpose of their D/s relationship is to spice up their sex life.

However, the main question your Dominant has about you is this: are you submissive material? These are the hallmarks of a good submissive:

- Willingness
- Obedience
- Eagerness to serve

The time a Dominant spends training his sub will vary, but the average time is one month. At the beginning of this training period, the Dominant may place a training collar around his sub's neck to symbolize that she has entered her training. Some also choose to use a training contract that outlines a training time of ninety days, six months, or even one year. At the end of the training period, the Dominant may place a permanent collar around his sub's neck to symbolize that she's successfully completed her training period. This collar is usually more of a formal one, but that doesn't mean it needs to be worn by the sub at all times. She may choose to only wear it in the house or during BDSM sex.

My Dominant placed a training collar around my neck after I agreed to submit to him, and he accepted my submission. This process didn't happen overnight; in our particular case, it took place in steps. First, we spent a period of time getting to know each other out of bed to see whether or not we were compatible; then, we had a couple of sessions of regular sex before my Dominant gradually began to introduce small signs of domination that I picked up on right away. At that point, he clearly explained what he was going to do to me in our first "scene," which would include a blindfold and necktie for the gentle binding of my wrists. It was after this introductory scene that he asked if I would like to submit to him. He then explained that it was a big responsibility for him to accept my submission and wanted to know why I wanted to submit to him before deciding. At that point, I told him that it was because I didn't know any other way to be, and despite my hasty agreement, he still insisted on giving me a couple of days to think it over before accepting my submission.

Soon afterward, my Dominant returned from a business trip where he had made a side trip to a sex shop to purchase a training collar for me and a couple of other sex toys. "This is your training collar," he announced as he placed it around my neck. He then told me that I was to call him Sir in the bedroom and other parts of the house when the situation dictated it. Afterward, he showed me the other two sex toys before explaining what he would do to me in the next scene in a step-by-step format.

We also discussed our limits and found that they were the same; therefore, we decided that a detailed written contract wouldn't be necessary. At that point, my Dominant gave me my first written training assignment, and over the next four weeks, he proceeded to provide me with several more. These exercises are great intimacy-building tools designed to allow the Dominant to get into his submissive's head. They allow the Dominant to get to know his submissive's innermost desires, fantasies, weaknesses, and fears in a safe environment—on the page. Here's a list of sample training assignments a Dominant might use:

Training Assignment #1:

Describe to me in a scene how you wish to be dominated.

Training Assignment #2:

Describe to me a fantasy that you've always had.

Training Assignment #3:

List ten scenes that you'd like to do in bed.

Training Assignment #4:

Tell me what you love most about the way I dominate you.

Training Assignment #5:

Tell me what you love most about submitting to me.

You might want to find a submissive training notebook online or just purchase an ordinary spiral notebook to complete your training assignments. If your handwriting isn't the finest, you could also choose to write them on the computer. This training notebook may also be used as your submissive's journal that you can use to express yourself and work out your issues. Just remember that the training notebook will need to be shown to your Dominant, while the submissive's journal may or may not be shown to him. A submissive's journal is usually the property of the submissive; however, this should all be negotiated, so there are no surprises.

Written assignments are one part of a submissive's training; another part will involve tasks. Whether these tasks will involve domestic service or not will depend on whether you and your Dominant have a "lifestyle" D/s relationship that extends outside of the bedroom. This should not be confused with a 24/7 D/s relationship, where a submissive remains in service to her Dominant twenty-four hours a day. This is deemed extremely hard to achieve, as it may not be possible due to outside commitments such as work and family.

A sample task that you might be given by your Dominant might be a simple one, such as an order to shave your private area, or it might be a challenging one, such as a drive to the store while wearing a butt plug beneath your skirt. My Dominant once threatened me with the latter but then changed his mind. He often uses this tactic to maximize excitement, and it works quite well. There's nothing wrong with having no limits as long as it's confined to the erotic imagination.

But what about the assignment of tasks in the bedroom? Will the purchase of BDSM toys be left solely up to your Dominant? Will you be allowed to speak in bed or make requests? He may prefer that you don't speak at all during sex or prefer that you only speak when spoken to. He may also wish that you only use the phrases, "Yes, Sir," and, "Thank you, Sir." You will notice that, "No, Sir," is not one of the phrases. That's because, in the world of BDSM, we don't use the word no; we use what's called a "top word" or "safe word."

The decision of whether to use a "safe word" is an important one that should be made during the initial negotiations between you and your Dominant. The word you agree upon shouldn't be one that might come up during BDSM sex, such as vagina. It should clearly express that the submissive has reached some limit when it comes to pain or humiliation. One might choose a word such as "red" or "giraffe." What's important is that your Dominant immediately stop whatever he's doing once he hears you say the stop word. This is vital to the development of trust within your D/s relationship.

After all, if a submissive goes far enough into "sub-space" during play, she can injure herself without knowing it. The intoxicating feelings of sub-space within the world of BDSM can vary greatly from sub to sub, just as some are more receptive to hypnosis than others. While some may experience a floating feeling, others may enter a near trance-like state. But when the sub's system stops producing morphine-like drugs, she may feel a drop in temperature, exhaustion, incoherence, and incoordination. This is referred to as "sub-drop" in BDSM, which is why aftercare is important.

Once your Dominant feels you have passed the training contract phase, he may want you to acquire skills in areas such as the following:

- Dance
- A sport
- Formal entertainment
- Cooking
- Massage therapy
- Small business management

I'm now going to show you a day in my life as a trained submissive. It doesn't at all mean that it should be a day in your life. Do what makes you happy.

Typical Sunday:

9:00 am I wake up and very carefully move back the covers so as not to awaken my Dominant. Then I put on a satin robe and make the coffee, blending the exact number of scoops between 2 flavors of coffee grounds that he likes.

9:45 am I serve my Dominant bacon and an omelet made with rosemary that I ground in a mortar and pestle the way my Dominant likes it. I also sauté his mushrooms and spinach in the herbs before pouring on the eggs. Then we have breakfast together.

10:30 am I wash the breakfast dishes while wearing the white, frilly apron that my Dominant purchased for me.

11:00 am I change into lingerie, and my Dominant takes me back to bed for BDSM morning sex.

11:45 am I may massage my Dominant's calves and feet on the massage table if they're feeling especially sore.

12:00 pm I shower and shave my complete body the way my Dominant prefers it.

1:00 pm I put on my tennis skirt and top and my Dominant and I play tennis.

2:15 pm I serve my Dominant a lunch of leftovers from dining out.

3:00 pm I put on a skimpy maid outfit and throw our clothes in the washer after carefully cleaning out my Dominant's pockets.

3:15 pm I file my nails so as not to scratch my Dominant during sex or massage.

3:35 pm I place our clothes in the dryer.

3:45 pm I grab a carryall for cleaning products and clean the bathrooms while wearing my maid outfit.

4:30 pm I get the clothes out of the dryer and fold them.

5:00 pm I put my apron back on and begin cooking a gourmet dinner for my Dominant and me.

7:00 pm I serve my Dominant dinner, and we eat together.

8:00 pm I do the dinner dishes in my maid outfit.

9:00 pm I watch TV or a film with my Dominant.

10:30 pm I change into jeans, and my Dominant and I walk 1.5 miles.

11:00 pm I change into different lingerie and give my Dominant a full or partial body massage on the table, then I wipe off the lotion from his body with a towel from the towel warmer.

11:30 pm My Dominant and I have BDSM sex.

❧ Chapter 5 ❧

Conditioning

My Stepfather, the Sadist — Gregor is from Liverpool in North West England. He speaks with a British accent, has mutton chop sideburns, a thick, dark mustache, and a clean-shaven chin. He's had the sideburns since the early 1970s when mutton chops were the height of fashion. At that time, they displayed class, intellect, and masculinity above other competing males. Incidentally, they were also popular in the porn industry.

There's a curved palm tree in the front yard of Gregor's house that stands out like a phallic symbol. The backyard is surrounded by a thick wall of rubber tree plants and pink and yellow hibiscus flowers. A small, concrete deck sports an umbrella table and leaves just enough room for a folding chaise lounge chair that Gregor likes to use for nude sunbathing. He's very proud of the all-over dark tan he's able to achieve despite Brits being known for their ghostly pallor. He also keeps strict watch of his waistline and weighs himself methodically each morning.

Another source of Gregor's pride comes from the Florida room he's decorated and equipped with a full bar made of black leather. His large Doberman Pinscher, Baine, often curls up in one of the two matching black leather saucer chairs in the corner. The bright orange shag carpet in the

Florida room contrasts nicely and offsets the rest of the carpet in the house, which is avocado green. The two colors also prevail in the kitchen, just as they do in many other households. But Gregor plays by his own rules.

The first rule of the house is made known to his wife, Laura, in a strict fashion. Gregor makes it clear that he's a nudist and that they're now a nudist family who will not wear clothes in the house unless it happens to be cold—a rare event in South Florida. And even when the temperature drops now and then on a random day in the winter, she's to ask permission of Gregor to wear clothes. They'll also become members of a nudist colony in Fort Pierce, Florida, called Sun Gardens that they'll frequently visit in their RV.

* * * * *

Keeping someone in the nude is one of many conditioning or brainwashing techniques that's meant to reduce their ability to think critically or independently. It's also meant to change their attitudes, values, and beliefs while allowing the introduction of new thoughts and ideas into their minds. Because of this, you're going to want to be very careful about the Dominant you choose. You'll want to take a look at the life he leads. Does he make decisions on a whim? Does he take advice from anyone at face value without considering the source? Does he save for the future or spend his last dollar on a beer?

And how about you? Will you still be able to maintain enough of your critical thinking to know whether your Dominant is crossing boundaries of a legal or ethical nature? What if he asks you to carry his drugs in a place that no one but him should search before boarding a plane? And would you be able to speak up to him if he did? The law doesn't recognize sub or slave mentality as a defense, so you'd better have a strong sense of identity before undergoing conditioning that's meant to break it down. This includes being conscious of your strengths and weaknesses and the way you operate internally.

It's also vital that your Dominant respect women, so you'll want to listen closely to the way he speaks about them. Are they all bitches and whores to him? Does he trash them behind their backs or to their faces? How about his views on marriage? Does he believe it to be a bad business proposition or an unnecessary and dying institution? You may not wish to get married, but his views on the subject may shed some light on his partnership skills.

Speaking of women, how's your Dominant's relationship with his mother? Does he spend time with her either in person or on the phone? Is his family valuable to him? How does he treat them? How do they treat him? These questions extend to friends, as well. You can tell a lot about a person by the close friends they've chosen, so take a good hard look at them. Are they manipulative? Irresponsible? Thrill seeking? Chances are, your Dominant has a lot of the same qualities, or he wouldn't be relating to them.

If you find any of the answers to these questions disturbing, then you shouldn't enter into a D/s relationship with your Dominant because one or both of you has a lot of work to do on themselves first. And while it's true that life's a journey that causes us to grow through our experiences, we should never give up our power to anyone who's likely to abuse it. We should also never give up our ability to anyone without checks and balances in place, which is where a D/s contract comes in.

Whatever kind of relationship you currently have with your partner is going to be amplified by BDSM. For example, if you have an abusive relationship, it's going to get even more abusive, and if you have a healthy relationship, it's going to get even healthier. This is why it's vitally important that you consider points such as these first and be honest with yourself. Now let's take a look at some of the rest of the conditioning techniques out there.

HYPNOSIS - This technique induces a high state of suggestibility in the submissive. It usually involves the Dominant using a firm but even voice while the submissive stares at a still object, such as a lit candle.

ISOLATION - This technique induces the loss of reality by physical separation from family, friends, and society as a whole.

REMOVAL OF PRIVACY - This technique involves achieving the loss of the ability to evaluate logically by preventing private contemplation.

DRESS CODE - This technique involves the removal of individuality by demanding conformity to a dress code.

REJECTION OF OLD VALUES - This technique involves accelerating the acceptance of a new lifestyle by constantly denouncing former beliefs and values.

METACOMMUNICATION - This technique involves the implementation of subliminal messages by stressing specific keywords or phrases.

UNCOMPROMISING RULES - This technique induces disorientation and regression by soliciting agreement to seemingly simple rules which regulate mealtimes, bathroom breaks, etc.

CONTROLLED APPROVAL - This technique involves rewarding and punishing.

NO QUESTIONS - This technique accomplishes the automatic acceptance of beliefs by discouraging questions.

❧ Chapter 6 ☙

The History of BDSM

Laura heads up the driveway and makes her way over to the door, but just as she lifts her hand to reach for the knob, it occurs to her that she's not been given a key to Gregor's house. Sure enough, the door's locked. Laura turns around with a furrowed brow and heads over to the wooden gate on the right side of the house. This, at least, is unlocked. She glances briefly at the side door to the small garage before making her way to the umbrella table, which provides a bit of shade from the relentless sun. After setting her purse down on the tile tabletop, Laura slides down onto one of the concrete benches and ponders what to do next. Several minutes go by before she notices a loquat tree in the corner of the yard. It will provide her with sustenance while she waits for Gregor to come home, which will not be for another hour.

"Gregor, I don't have a key," Laura informs Gregor upon his return. "May I have a house key?"

Gregor thinks about this for a moment as he unlocks the door. "No, not for the first week. And make sure you take off your clothes when you get inside." He then goes off to the bedroom. Laura follows him and pulls off her shorts, top, and panties just as he's said. They're now nudists in Gregor's house, and his rules are to be followed at all times.

"If I can't have a key, then what am I supposed to do when I get home?" Laura asks him.

"You can wait in the garage. I'll leave the side door to the garage unlocked, and you can wait in there until I get home," Gregor replies, satisfied with his plan.

"But it's dark in there and hot," she whines.

"Well, too bad. You're not getting a key to the house until your first week of training is up," he orders. *"Now go prepare dinner."*

* * * * *

The definition of bondage is the state of being a slave. BDSM has long roots in history; it didn't just crop up overnight. Over the last century, it's become a lifestyle with its own protocol. Some people believe Alfred Kinsey was the first to use S/M in the 1940s. Still, the term BDSM wasn't coined until 1969 in an essay by Kinsey's collaborator and anthropologist, Paul Gebhard, titled "Fetishism and Sadomasochism." Gebhard was the first to explore BDSM as a cultural phenomenon; however, many ancient cultures depicted sexual acts with sadomasochistic elements.

BDSM has its roots in Mesopotamia, where gods and monsters are said to have ruled over human subjects. Inanna is the ancient Mesopotamian goddess associated with sex, war, justice, and political power. Some of the first stories in ancient history involved sexual acts of dominance and submission. They were centered around Inanna, who worshiped her own vagina and forced men to bow to her in submission. She's also said to have whipped her subjects as they danced for her, enticing them into sexual frenzies.

BDSM also has its roots in Ancient Greece. During the ninth century, whipping was used as an initiation rite in a religious cult in Sparta dedicated to the goddess Artemis Orthia. Priestesses would oversee the flagellation of young men. Whipping for sexual pleasure was also taking place inside The Tomb of Whipping. The focus wasn't on the physical act of sex, however. In the *History of Sexuality*, Michael Foucault wrote about how sex served as a method of initiation into learning in Greece.

Inside Italy's "Tomb of The Floggings," a wall painting depicts a woman getting whipped by two men during an erotic tryst. The tomb, which was built around the fifth century BCE, is believed to be dedicated to Dionysus, a god associated with debauchery. In Pompeii, wall frescoes inside the "Villa of Mysteries" show a winged "Whipstress" who supposedly initiated women into the secret cult of "Mysteries" through techniques like bondage and flagellation. Whipping may well have been more than just an act of punishment. Perhaps it was also a sacred or sexual act at one time.

In Rome's early days, men (but not women) who were condemned to crucifixion were scourged beforehand. This meant they were stripped naked, tied to a post, and flogged across the back, buttocks, and legs by soldiers. There were also Roman Catholic monks who practiced self-flagellation. The church permitted flagellation to "purge oneself of sin" to avoid sickness during the Black Plague.

In Sparta, priestesses would whip men to make them more masculine. Greeks and Romans associated the whipping of the buttocks with fertility. In England, thieves were flogged near the scene of their crime, and in America, slaves were flogged.

The Indian *Kama Sutra*, one of the oldest books about sex and sexual positions, is also the oldest known guide to ethically incorporating torture into sex. The book was written in Sanskrit sometime between 400 BCE and 300 CE. It's also about a lot more than just sex. The *Kama Sutra* is actually a guide to existence and happiness, which is believed to have a lot to do with sexuality and eroticism. The book uses poetry and prose to describe many philosophical ideas about love and life. It includes relationship advice, power dynamics in marriage, and ways to partake in what we would call BDSM today. There's a chapter on consensual slapping and another called "Types of Scratching with the Nails." Four types of hitting during sex are said to be permissible, but only with people who find such activities "joyful." The *Kama Sutra* teaches men and women to respect each other, as the goal is liberation from this world. This is to be done through the basic principles of trust, communication, and consent.

In the late 1700s, the Marquis de Sade published *120 Days of Sodom*. This book included group sex, humiliation, beatings, forced orgasms, and role play. Perhaps it caused the focus of BDSM to shift from being about honesty and trust to control and sexual gratification.

BDSM really became known, however, in the twentieth century following World War I. People looking for fun and a new way of life began creating clubs where they could be free to express their alternative sexuality. The clubs were eventually destroyed by Hitler and Fascism, even though some of the patrons were fascists. The practice of BDSM then went underground along with the publication of "sex" magazines in the 1940s and 1950s that featured role models like Bettie Page. The latex, leather, high heels, and corsets she wore helped create the modern look of BDSM. Miss Page is also partly responsible for the sexual revolution of the 1960s. She encouraged women to embrace their sexuality through the role of either submissive or dominatrix. This was when BDSM began to shift from the underground to a budding artistic movement.

Born Submissive

Part II

ဆ Chapter 7 ⌒

Punishment

Dinner choices, like everything else in Gregor's house, are made by Gregor. He decides what we eat, on which night of the week we eat it, and on which night of the week he and Laura eat out. For example, Monday night is knockwurst and cabbage night, Tuesday night is liver and onions night, and on Friday night, he and Laura go to Gentleman Jim's for steak. Unless, of course, Laura disobeys him. Then Gentleman Jim's is held over her head like a carrot on a stick that she won't be getting.

And then there's the dog.

Baine is a full-grown, male, black Doberman Pinscher that stands about two and a half feet high, weighs about 75 pounds, and does not like blacks. The sight of our black mailman sets him off on an angry barking spree each day that lasts for several minutes. The man dreads whenever he has to drop off any packages for us on our front step, where he has to lower his head towards the menacing sounds coming from just behind the door. He then hurries back out of our yard and down the street.

In the early days of this first house, I enjoy Baine. Gregor shows me how he gets him to lay down by placing his hand on his long nose on its way down to the floor. I try to do it myself a few times but only achieve marginal success, as I'm only four feet tall. Then one day, I see Baine run into the kitchen and rise against the counter with his front paws so he can peer out the window. In that position, I notice how easy it would be for him to tower over me. I also notice that he has sharp claws that scrape against the cabinets on the way down. Baine has been trained to kill upon Master's command.

During dinner, Baine remains curled up on the floor of the kitchen in the corner. He knows better than to beg at the table, for Gregor is just as swift with punishment for the dog as he is with Laura. He always insists that Baine heel before going out for a walk and is quick with several leash lashes against his ribs whenever he disobeys.

Baine often jumps up on my bed to look out the window whenever he hears the slightest noise outside. One time the sound of a possum scurrying around in the attic drives him so insane that Gregor has to set a trap to catch the animal. The sound of its little claws on the wood sends Baine bounding from room to room in a frantic attempt to see where the noise is coming from. Gregor finally manages to trap the possum. Then he gets back to training Baine and Laura.

* * * * *

My earliest memory of a spanking dates back to when I was five years old. It was actually more of a fear of getting spanked by a babysitter watching both the neighbor boy and me. She had taken the neighbor boy into his mother's bedroom and made loud spanking sounds with a belt, so I would believe he was getting spanked. Each time the belt cracked, I heard the boy yowl. Then she had told me that I was next, which caused me to burst into tears. "Shouldn't only boys get spanked?" I whined. I was a girl, and I was younger than the neighbor boy. It wasn't fair. I remember telling my mother about the threat when she came home, but she'd just brushed it off as a joke. I, however, hadn't found it amusing at all.

When I received my first spanking as an adult, I found it both provocative and arousing. My dominant had ordered me to bend over his knees so that my head had almost touched the floor. How humiliating and yet thrilling it had been at the same time. Each strike of his hand had left a red mark on my ass cheek, yet he clearly hadn't cared one bit. He'd even made me count all nineteen blows. Nineteen!

Punishment can be administered for either admonishment or erotic pleasure, but there will often be overlap. The reason for this has to do with how the body and brain deal with pain and the psychological aspects of dominance and submission. One of the factors is dopamine, which is present in the body during both pain and pleasure. The body also releases endorphin, serotonin, melatonin, epinephrine, and norepinephrine. These chemicals all help re-balance our bodies whenever we feel physical or emotional stress, such as with exercise. The pain can also become addictive with the sub experiencing intoxication, craving and withdrawal, and tolerance.

The punishment of flogging done in ancient times was very different from the BDSM flogging of today. There were no contracts, no safe words, and no aftercare. In other words, the consent was missing. The goal was not sub-space euphoria but torture and humiliation. Slaves who escaped from their masters were used as a warning to other slaves through public floggings or crucifixions.

When considering whether you will consent to be punished by your Dominant, you should ask yourself the following questions: First, do you trust your Dominant enough to allow him to administer punishment to you? If not, then you shouldn't be in a D/s relationship with him at all, as trust is a crucial element of BDSM. Second, how's your pain tolerance? If the answer is low, would you be willing to train yourself to take more pain? Third, what kind of punishment are you willing to endure? A light flogging or lashes with a belt or whip? Counting down lets the sub know when the pain will end, which is helpful. Of course, the punishment should always be negotiated up front, and you can always change your mind if you find the pain non-arousing or unbearable. Personally, I love the quickness with which my Dominant reacts to an infraction by me. The immediate order to drop my pants for a spanking tends to reduce me to wet mush just as much as when he immediately rips an article of my clothing at his whim.

During the course of a D/s relationship, the first form of punishment may arise when the sub tries to test the boundaries of her Dominant's rules. Perhaps she's too tired for sex one night and decides to find out how this will go over with him. Everyone gets tired sometimes. In fact, her Dominant may even be tired and welcome a break that night. Yet, he must remain consistent about enforcing his rules. This may be when a Dominant chooses to use the "cold shoulder" approach. In this approach, the Dominant simply agrees to let the sub go to sleep; however, he does not kiss her goodnight, cuddle her, or do any of the things he usually does. Instead, he ignores her while he reads or watches TV. Then the following morning, he admonishes the sub for being disrespectful to him.

Another form of punishment besides the "cold shoulder" and the spanking may be implemented when the sub hasn't technically broken a rule; she's simply done something that the Dominant doesn't like. When this happens, your Dominant's punishment of choice may be anal penetration. However, this will not be done in an especially erotic way. This may still make for a very arousing experience for the sub, but it will also be done in a way that will stay with her for a long time to come.

On the flip side of this (literally), the Dominant may pin his sub down on the bed with his body while strapping the tie from her robe through her teeth. The amount of pressure he may exert will be his own personal choice and may leave temporary marks on her face cheeks rather than her ass. The sub may find this form of "double-pinning" extremely arousing.

One of the more subtle (yet not so subtle) forms of psychological punishment involves viewing torture pornography. In this case, the Dominant may put on a clip that reflects his level of annoyance with his sub. For example, it may feature a sexy female wearing a ball gag in her mouth. Another one may feature a woman tied up by way of Japanese rope bondage. And if the Dominant is extremely annoyed with his sub, he may put on a clip of a female screaming while being pulled around by her hair.

Now I'd like to discuss something that I haven't seen expounded upon very much in other BDSM books: pain tolerance. Occasionally an author will attempt to advise on how to deal with the pain that can sometimes accompany BDSM (remember, pain is optional and should always be negotiated upfront). However, I haven't seen much more than the breathing techniques mentioned. They tell you that you should breathe through the pain, which is excellent advice.

Breathing through the pain will help you get through the level that your body is currently able to tolerate—but that's all. Athletes will tell you that you must train your nervous system to take the pain. How do runners condition their bodies to run farther? They train themselves to run farther each day. And how do weightlifters train their bodies to lift more weight? They train themselves to lift more weight each day. Each activity comes with pain. My suggestion to you is that you get into even better physical condition by participating in a sport you like. This will not only increase your pain tolerance but will also increase your endurance during sex. Your Dominant will not only appreciate the new level of fitness that you've achieved, but you'll be able to handle that spanking on the inside of your thighs like a pro. Not your thing? No problem. You can always opt for a flogger from the BDSM Toys chapter in the next section. Remember, BDSM is like an actor's wardrobe—only wear what you like and be comfortable in your own skin.

❧ Chapter 8 ❧

Journaling

"So, how's your new husband treating Deanna?" my dad asks Laura one day soon after we've moved into Gregor's house.

"Fine. She likes him," she says into the avocado green rotary phone that hangs from the wall in the kitchen.

"How do you know? Did you hear that from her, or from him?" my dad pries.

"I can just tell," Laura replies. Then she hears a click. And some breathing. Now every time my dad calls, Gregor sneaks into the bedroom, picks up the phone, and listens in on their conversation. Afterward there's always a serious debriefing, and she better not have said anything he doesn't like, or punishment will be administered.

Gregor's punishment comes in several different forms that usually involve more of a lifestyle change for Laura than an immediate correction. For example, if she displeases him, her weekly allowance gets decreased, but not for any specified period of time, just until further notice, which usually comes once Gregor is finally pleased. Other forms of punishment involve food, which led to the addition of liver and onions to the weekly menu. If there's one thing I hate more than eating liver, it's the stench it gives off while being cooked. It's one smell Baine craves and I loathe. He gets his own serving of boiled chicken livers whenever we dine on beef liver. It's like a private celebration for Baine's Master that he enjoys along with his dog.

* * * * *

Journals have been used for centuries to document our ancestors' personal history. They've helped us understand a great deal about life in the past and the people who lived during that time. Scientific studies have proven that writing about our feelings provides us with many mental and physical benefits. A UCLA study found that journaling dampens activity in the brain that results in us feeling happier and regulates emotions more effectively. Researchers have shown us that journaling can strengthen a critical part of the immune system and decrease the symptoms of illnesses such as rheumatoid arthritis and asthma. Another study has demonstrated that writing about our feelings can make us less likely to become ill and cushion us from stressors and traumas. Writing also helps us to heal.

It can be very hard for a submissive to bring up issues with her Dominant when they arise. After all, she's supposed to want what her Dominant wants, right? But what about the times when she doesn't? What about the times when he's crossed over a boundary and hurt her feelings? Speaking to your Dominant in anger and forgetting your place is a punishable offense in BDSM. However, holding in such emotions will only cause them to well up and overflow in much the same manner. This is why it's much better to allow yourself a reflective period before expressing your feelings. Speaking in anger without thinking can cause a breakdown of respect. This is how cracks develop in the relationship; therefore, it's much better to defuse your anger by first expressing your thoughts in a journal. That way, you can sleep on it and reread it the next day once your anger has subsided.

Sometimes I spend weeks writing about a particularly painful issue that I'm having with my Dominant. Each time I pick my journal back up, the problem becomes clearer to me until I've found just the right words that I need. There's also a feeling of relief that I didn't send my letter to him prematurely before adequately stating my case. This is how effective communication is achieved, so take the time to do it right.

You don't need to spend a lot of money on your journal, but you should make it fun. There are both hard and soft-bound versions online; however, a simple pocket black spiral for your purse will work just as well. It helps to have one at your fingertips when you're needing to vent about a particular issue. Perhaps writing the words: "I will be patient with _____" for an entire page will be therapeutic at times or even listing inspirational quotes. The point is to develop a routine for venting and releasing the built-up tension that inevitably comes with any relationship.

In addition to a pocket spiral for the rough drafts of my thoughts, I've also chosen the computer as a method of communication to my Dominant. My letters to him all have three main elements in common:

- The date
- A graphic header at the top
- A graphic footer at the bottom

Which graphics have I chosen, you ask? Well, that's personal, but you can be assured that my Dominant likes them. I know because I asked him. I also have an electronic folder on my computer where I save them. Creating a formal template for my letters helps set the tone for respectful and sophisticated messages. My thoughts will then be expressed in a clear and focused manner. My Dominant can also look back on them and reread them if necessary, which he often does.

And what goes into those letters? Well, that's also a private matter, but the format isn't, so I will gladly expound upon it here. In the first paragraph of my letter, I always point out one of my Dominant's positive qualities or actions. I also end on a positive note so that the entry reflects our relationship's positive nature while pointing out a particular issue that we need to (and will) work out. I resolved early on that failure would not be an option for us, which forces us to work out our problems. I did this because I feel it's often too easy for people to give up on each other when they keep this option available. This doesn't mean that my method is in any way foolproof; it's just a mindset that I keep.

Many subs (including me) may find it extremely difficult and perhaps even impossible to verbally express discontent to their Dominant. Their heart may be beating out of their chest in fear, and the words may enter their head but never leave by way of their mouth. Because of this dilemma, I feel it's absolutely crucial for a sub to keep a journal. Over time the sub may get better at expressing herself verbally, but the journal will definitely be a tool that helps her do so. It can be a critical line of communication between a Dominant and his sub.

❧ Chapter 9 ❦

Mind Games

The new brown and beige motorhome that Gregor purchased takes up the entire driveway. I invite my friend, Robin, over to see it. I show her the overhead loft bed, and we sing the disco song "Boogie Nights" together and dance around. I have no idea what a nudist colony is, but I'm about to find out.

Sun Gardens Nudist Colony in Fort Pierce, Florida, boasts that it's the most naturally tropical naturist resort in the United States and possibly one of its friendliest communities. Nudity is expected at Sun Gardens, where they promote healthful living and a family-friendly environment. Everyone is welcome to enjoy the volleyball, tennis, and petanque courts, as well as kayaking, swimming pool, sauna, spa, playground, and nature trails. Sun Gardens offers a full range of accommodations from deluxe cabin rentals, to full-hookup R.V. sites, to primitive tenting. There, one can experience a friendly, natural paradise where one can enjoy the freedom of feeling the sunshine and water all over them.

"Wait, I need to pack a bag before we go," Laura says as she looks over uneasily at Gregor.

"If you want to pack a bag, you can pack a bag," Gregor shrugs.

Laura hurries inside and throws some shorts, tops, and bikinis into a duffle bag. "Okay, I'm ready," she says as she steps onto the metal steps of the R.V. Suddenly, Gregor snatches the bag from her hand and carries it back into the house.

A few moments later, he returns. "I said you could pack a bag, not bring it with us. I told you this is a nudist colony. There are no clothes allowed," he orders as he climbs up into the R.V.

It's going to be a long ride.

I settle onto one of the orange twill bench seats by the dining table and watch Baine pace restlessly back and forth inside his confined quarters. Occasionally, he stops to pant in the heat and displays his large, dirty fangs. Eventually, he curls up against the back sofa's wooden base for a nap. I know he'll be allowed to stay inside the R.V. once we get to the camp. I, however, will not be allowed.

* * * * *

Carl Jung called the unknown dark side of the personality the shadow. He believed that within this shadow lurked everything we have forbidden ourselves to be aware of, such as shame, family secrets, and trauma. Perhaps BDSM takes us into our shadow, which then leads to healing. Somewhere along the way, however, there will be mind games.

My favorite mind games tend to begin with my Dominant taking me by the hair, pulling my head back, forcing me on my knees, and telling me what I can and cannot do after asking, "Are you my sex toy?" I long to be told what to do by my Dominant and want to give him complete control. I'm also aroused by the fear of being punished for forgetting to ask permission or doing a task incorrectly. Even receiving the words in a text makes me drip down my thighs.

Once again, it's crucial that you trust your Dominant enough to allow him to get into your head and play on your fears and insecurities. It's also vital that he recognize and act on any psychological triggers that cause you trauma. For example, if any words bring continued resistance from you, then he's crossed a line with that particular mind game and should stop.

During the training assignment phase of your BDSM relationship, you might have disclosed some of your personal history to your Dominant to allow him access to your thoughts. Exploring your past is necessary, but dodging the landmines can be tricky. If your Dominant's going to exploit any of your personal information, that should first be negotiated. For example, if you've always felt that your calves are too skinny, should your Dominant be able to degrade you about them? That depends on whether or not you find the degradation acceptable. If you feel the comments help you become comfortable with your body the way it is, then your Dominant should degrade away. If not, then you should let your Dominant know and he should stop.

Aftercare is a time to clear up any residual effects from the mind games. This is the period after a BDSM scene when the Dominant holds and cares for his sub. He should also make sure she's kept warm. Some feel that this should also be a time for your Dominant to assure you that you're still attractive and loved by him. After all, he may have just seen how low you're willing to go for him. If that's the case, you may need some raising back up.

❧ Chapter 10 ❧

Bondage & Humiliation

"We're here," Gregor announces from the captain's chair of his R.V. I watch as he rotates in the driver's seat with his tanned legs.

"Where's Baine? He needs to go for a pee, and so do I," Gregor informs us as he steps down. "Well? What are you waiting for? Get those clothes off. Let's go have some fun, shall we?"

I do what I'm told and strip off my clothes, fully intending to return later and put them back on. I slowly fold them and set them on the bench seat, where I've spent the last hour trying to figure a way out of my predicament. Unfortunately, there's no getting out of it. Soon I'll be thrust out of the motorhome and thrown into the Florida jungle.

My first glimpse of the nudist colony reveals several tall posts that resemble telephone poles. Giant green tarps have been strung up between them to separate the "nudies" from the outside world. I'm struck by how makeshift it all seems. This is it? I think. After hearing all of the hype about how the entire planet should be carousing around in their birthday suits, it seems as if this little section of South Florida is hiding its hedonism. And rightfully so—nudism venues are few and far between. To the rest of the world, nudists are heathens.

"Go on. Go explore and have some fun," Gregor urges me as he scoots me out of the R.V. "We'll see you back here for lunch at one."

I head reluctantly toward one of the tarps and stare back at Laura just in time to see her wave. Beyond the tarp is a large sand volleyball court full of naked bodies. Men and women jump with sagging breasts and flopping bellies. They punch at the ball and half-heartedly try to send it over the net. I can hear their yips and awws as I hurry past them with my head down. Who are these people, and how did they all get here? I wonder.

The pool is next. The water has a greenish tint to it and is full of naked people on floats. Nude children frolic along its sides while their parents bask in the sun on multi-colored towels. I watch a fat man rub suntan lotion on his wife's plump shoulders. Beyond the pool to the right is a hot tub full of more nude patrons. I hurry past the melee and pull open a set of sliding glass doors. Inside it looks like a rec room with a worn, wooden floor. There's a pool table, a ping pong table, and a long folding table beneath a window.

"Lunch is at twelve-thirty," a middle-aged nude man announces to me when he sees me. "We're having hot dogs today." I nod and try to avoid looking at his genitals as I head out the back screen door.

* * * * *

In the 1500s, bondage and humiliation were practiced through the martial art Hojōjutsu, which is the art of rope restraint. Samurai bound prisoners using secret knots and elaborate rope configurations to keep them from escaping.

They were then paraded around while bound to humiliate them publicly. The intricate arrangements were quite complicated; therefore, they remained secretly guarded by individual clans. Interestingly, Hojōjutsu paved the way for Japanese erotic rope bondage or Shibari and Kinbaku. The art died out once Japan discovered handcuffs; however, it lives on in BDSM.

There are many forms of erotic humiliation, but the most common form tends to be verbal. Phrases such as "dirty slut," "sex toy," and "f*** doll" will trigger a sub's submissiveness and arouse her. Being told that the Dominant is only there to pleasure himself and that he doesn't care whether the sub is sexually satisfied can be arousing if the tactic is used sparingly. Using the tactic often would defeat the purpose of BDSM sex. The supremacy tactic where the sub is told that the Dominant is obviously more intelligent than her because he's male can also be arousing. BDSM, as you can see, isn't for everyone.

I happen to prefer the threat of exposure to public humiliation. I also don't like to walk around the house in the nude. My Dominant respects this request but still reserves the right to overrule it at any time. With the threat of exposure, my Dominant can go on endlessly about how he will tell my boss, my friends, or my mother just how horny I am. He won't really follow through with the exposure, but just the threat alone turns me on. He can reassure me of this during aftercare if he feels it's needed, but I trust him to make that call.

There's a point for me, however, where that trust could be tested. For example, would I ever agree to allow my Dominant to place me in a locked cage? How about a wooden box? I once read a book called *Perfect Victim: The True Story of the Girl in the Box* by Carla Norton and Christine McGuire. This is the story about a young hitchhiker named Colleen Stan, who's kidnapped by a man and kept inside a homemade wooden box during much of the day and night. The man had a wife who "couldn't handle the pain," so Colleen was abducted to take his whippings instead. Whenever he yelled the word "attention," she was to strip under an archway and hold her hands above her head for this purpose. Around her neck was a thick black collar with an "S" pendant that stood for sub.

I found myself thinking about this story for days afterward. What would it be like to spend hours at a time locked inside a box? Surely it would be hot in there, but what about the boredom alone? I'm probably a person who'd fare better than a lot of others if I were ever to be locked inside a prison cell simply because I love to read and write. But what if I couldn't even do either of those things? And what about being away from the bathroom for hours at a time? Colleen didn't seem to fare well with that one in the book.

Her kidnapper also kept her strapped to a rack for hours at a time, which had most likely been hard on her circulation. What would've been going through her mind during that time? I wondered. She wanted to escape initially, but over time, the situation became familiar to her and felt like home. Still, could I ever accept a box as my home for hours at a time? No, I definitely could not. That would be a hard limit for me, which is one of the many reasons I'm not a slave.

ও Chapter 11 ಣ

Devaluation

The nudist colony's resort roads are made of packed sand, but there are also plenty of grassy areas and soft pine needle-coated paths. Many of the permanent residents grow tropical flowers and fruits such as jackfruit and mango. There are also camping and travel trailer areas located just inside some of the Florida jungle's natural openings, and vegetation is everywhere.

I trample past several mailboxes and mobile homes that sit behind picket fences, thinking how odd they all appear. The community seems fake, like a temporary camp that's pretending to be a neighborhood.

Later that afternoon, I find myself down by the cypress swamp watching people maneuver in canoes. I gratefully discover that the swamp provides shade from the hot Florida sun due to all of the leather ferns, wax myrtle, and pond apple trees. The canoes are almost starting to look like fun until I realize that my backside is now severely sunburned. I know I need out of the heat.

When I return to the R.V., it dawns on me that I'm an hour early for lunch. It's only twelve, yet I've been instructed not to return until one. My burned backside, however, says otherwise. I pull open the metal latch of the door and am greeted by Baine with his huge kisses. He's been lonely all day and is glad to see me. "Not now, boy," I tell him. I lock the door and head past Laura for the bathroom to examine my butt in the mirror. It's now tomato red.

I spend the next half hour lying on my stomach on the sofa and have just gotten up to get a drink when Laura and I hear someone trying to open the door. We glance over and hear them pull on the latch once again, then silence. A few moments later, Laura hears a voice above her head. "I had a feeling you'd be in here, you Pig! Get back outside. Now!"

Laura looks up and sees Gregor staring down at her from the pop-up vent on the roof of the R.V. "I can't. We're sunburned. We don't tan as well as you. I need to stay in here," she cries, already knowing it's in vain.

"Did you hear what I said? Get back out here now, or I'll make you stay out here all night," Gregor threatens. He then begins rattling the vent cover. "You haven't seen red yet until I get through with you! Do you hear me, you little Pig?"

Laura has no choice but to unlock the door. Gregor soon appears in the doorway larger than life. He's livid. She climbs onto the bench seat of the table and cowers there naked. Gregor lunges at her. He drags her by the arm into the open doorway, then lets go of her. "Get outside!" he orders. It's going to be a long weekend.

* * * * *

Erotic devaluation is about reducing the sub's worth or importance. It can come in either verbal or physical form, but the latter is often more extreme. Some verbal devaluation examples include objectification, such as when the sub is called a "sex toy," or ridiculing, such as when the sub is told her vagina's too wet to be of any use to her Dominant. Being made to ask permission to orgasm is another tactic a Dominant might use on his sub. He may even bring her to the edge and deny her request. Some examples of physical devaluation include orgasm on demand, forced orgasm (continued stimulation after orgasm has already been achieved), being used as furniture, being used as a human toilet, and being pulled around by a leash and collar.

The collar is very symbolic in the world of BDSM because it symbolizes ownership and commitment like a wedding ring. It also doesn't take a lot of time to implement, like a contract. BDSM collars are typically black leather with an O-ring and buckle, but they can consist of anything that can be worn around a submissive's neck. Some submissives like to wear a velvet ribbon or choker with or without a charm. That way, it can be worn discreetly to work or around extended family in the non-BDSM or "vanilla" world. Whether the collar should be worn at all times, like a wedding ring, will be up to the Dominant and the submissive. There are even collars that come with a padlock and key for that purpose. The more common practice is to only wear the collar inside the privacy of one's home.

Devaluation that's considered edgeplay can be psychologically devastating for a sub if not handled appropriately. For example, can you imagine wearing a paper bag over your head and being told that you're unattractive? It might sound distasteful to a lot of us, but there are some people out there who do it. Remember, there's a kink for everyone. Just make sure yours doesn't equal abuse.

So, how low are you willing to go for your Dominant? Would you drink water from a pet bowl? If so, is the water clean or dirty? Would you allow him to have sex with you against a window with no curtains? If so, does it overlook a busy street? You can see how circumstances can significantly alter the experience. This is another reason why negotiation is so important.

I love to bend to my Dominant's will. I live to serve and service him and love when he orders me to declare this as my "primary purpose." Begging is a turn-on. I also love when my Dominant makes fun of how aroused he's made me. "Look at you! What a dripping mess you are right now," he might say, or, "What a sloppy wet pussy you have." Either phrase said with exaggerated ridicule tends to put me in even worse shape.

Your Dominant may get good ideas about ways to devalue you from reading stories that you've written for him during your training assignments. He can also watch some of your favorite porn. Perhaps some scenes involve a woman in a short skirt being made to wear sticky notes on her that read "Office Slut," or maybe there's one that shows a man slapping a woman's face with his cock. There's nothing like a graphic example when it comes to letting your Dominant know what turns you on.

But what would a feminist think of all this? Once again, I'd like to add that labels are probably a silly and overly simplistic way of defining people. I'm not going to naively presume that all feminists are against BDSM or that the ones who are don't have any valid points of view. That would be closed-minded on my part. I will now give my opinion on a few of the common feminist debates about BDSM to show both sides of the argument.

1. **BDSM isn't always wholly consensual** - *Some feminists believe that women are sometimes pressured into participating in BDSM by their partners or that economic reasons are involved.* I wholeheartedly agree and acknowledge that these shouldn't be the reasons that women participate in BDSM.

2. **BDSM isn't about love and trust** - *Some feminists believe that those who participate in BDSM use love*

and trust to justify brutal and often dangerous acts of aggression. I partially agree that some people in the BDSM world abuse their power, just as some people in the rest of the world abuse their position of power.

3. **BDSM is immoral** - *Some feminists believe that those who participate in BDSM engage in immoral acts.* I'm afraid I have to disagree. Many who participate in BDSM are monogamous and what they do in the privacy of their bedroom is their business. It's incorrect to assume that everyone who engages in BDSM is either polyamorous or a sex worker.

4. **BDSM is not really sexually arousing** - *Some feminists believe that sexual arousal cannot be a reliable standard for BDSM because women often fake orgasms.* I'm afraid I have to disagree. D/s is an amplification of our natural primary purposes; therefore, it's inherently arousing.

5. **Society should aim for an equal world** - *some feminists believe that relations marked by inequalities in power, such as BDSM, should be avoided whenever possible.* I'm afraid I have to disagree. I believe that men and women have biological differences that define their primary purposes, which BDSM amplifies. A man's primary purpose is to compete, while a woman's primary purpose is to nurture. This doesn't mean that it should determine their purpose, however. We are all free to choose who we are.

❧ Chapter 12 ❧

Taskmaster

*The next house Gregor buys has four bedrooms and sits on half an acre of land away from the beach. This time he opts to put in a vaulted screened-in patio with a pool instead of a concrete deck. The BDSM is stepped up in the house, as well. Gregor now leaves notes on some of the fridge's food that read: Don't eat ****** (a derogatory name). These notes, Laura knows, are for her. Each night she's also ordered to clean both of the new stainless steel sinks with scouring powder after washing the dishes. When she's finished, Gregor inspects both sinks and drains to make sure they've been properly scrubbed.*

Occasionally Gregor allows Laura to have an out-of-town friend visit for a week, and she's allowed to wear clothes that week, but right before bed he orders her to take a shower. He then pulls her aside and tells her that while she's showering he might tell her friend that she never wears clothes in the house. It's a form of humiliation that raises a bit of fear in her each time that he might actually do it. Then the woman might not want to be her friend anymore. One time she loses a friend anyway when Baine corners the woman in a spare bedroom and humps her leg. The large dog also manages to push the mattress part of the way off the bed while doing it.

The friend refuses to visit ever again. Now Gregor has even more time to train Laura at the new house.

* * * * *

So, how complex will your domestic service tasks be? The answer will be in direct correlation with the complexity of your Dominant. For example, does he have sticky notes all over his desk? Does he have a pile of receipts and packing labels that he shreds weekly? If so, the tasks your Dominant assigns you might consist of cleaning out his fridge, polishing his shoes, picking up his dry cleaning, and more.

And will your Dominant be barking orders at you? A good Dominant will be firm but won't yell. This is because he'll be secure with himself and instructive with you. He might say, "I think I'm going to have you clean out the fridge now," or, "I'm going to have you polish my shoes." The tasks are really for both of you. You get to serve your Dominant, and he gets the benefit of your service. Your Dominant might also choose to reward you with sex or flowers.

A good Dominant should also be very observant and correct any infractions made by his sub. After all, she's putting a lot of time and effort into the tasks he's assigned her. She needs to know that her Dominant's rules are consistent and that he's putting just as much effort into their BDSM relationship as she is. He also has the responsibility of using his erotic imagination to direct the bedroom scenes. Therefore, laziness will not be a good trait of a Dominant.

Nor will laziness be a trait of a good sub. For the Dominant who is extremely particular about his food, a sub would fare well to view the preparation of his meals as a sports game. For example, the batter in a baseball game may only hit the ball thirty percent of the time, but this doesn't mean he should quit. Instead, he should be happy with the times that he hit the ball and ecstatic when he scores a home run. After all, aren't boredom and complacency some of the states we're trying to avoid by engaging in a D/s relationship in the first place? Embrace the challenge.

You should also get your training notebook out because you're going to want to make notes about your Dominant's needs and preferences. And don't underestimate the amount of detail you're going to want to note if you happen to have an extremely particular Dominant. Here's a list of some easily overlooked details about just his food alone:

1. What temperature does he like his meat cooked?

2. How cooked does he like his pasta?

3. How cooked does he like his vegetables?

4. Which vegetables does he like in his salad?

5. How thick does he like his cream sauces?

6. How brown does he like his toast?

7. Which wine does he enjoy with which food?

8. How much sour cream does he like in his beef stroganoff?

9. How much thyme does he want in his chicken marsala?

10. How thick does he like his meat sauce?

Unless you have a photographic memory, you'll find it helpful to keep notes about your Dominant's likes and dislikes. And try to remember the sports game analogy: stack the odds in your favor and don't be afraid to go back out to bat.

And a good Dominant should be noting his sub's needs and preferences in bed. Reading his sub's written training assignments will give him some hints, but the research shouldn't stop there. Does she like to have her wrists bound from behind while on her knees? Does she like to watch her Dominant dominate another woman? Does *she* want to dominate another woman?

Once a sub has been assigned a task by her Dominant, she's to continue the task on a regular basis. For example, if she's been instructed to take out the trash, she should do so each week. If she's been asked to make her Dominant's dental cleaning appointment, then she should make his follow-up appointments as well. Her Dominant shouldn't have to remind her about it constantly. Her primary purpose now is to make his life easier and to meet his needs.

There is one task, however, that a sub should give herself: Kegels. Kegels strengthen the pelvic floor muscles, which support the bladder, uterus, small intestine, and rectum. They can also improve the sexual experiences of both the Dominant and sub by improving sexual arousal and orgasms. You can do pelvic floor muscle training just about any time. I do them during my drive to work, which takes me half an hour. My version of pelvic floor muscle training, however, goes well beyond the standard one. I not only squeeze my pelvic floor muscles, but I also contract my abdomen and gluteal muscles for a count of ten and then release. The results have been astounding. Not only has control of my vaginal canal been increased, but the firmness of my abdomen and gluteal muscles has been noticeable as well. Trust me, no task will be appreciated by your Dominant more than this one.

Born Submissive

Part III

ಋ Chapter 13 ಜ

BDSM Toys

Laura's training often takes place behind the closed door of Gregor's bedroom, which is always kept very dark. The scorching Florida sun is never allowed to penetrate the windows' blackout drapes, but the room is hardly soundproof. Laughter occasionally filters in through the crack of the bedroom door amidst the smacks. Perhaps it's due to the large pink feather that's used for tickling bare skin.

A cat o' nine tails is also mentioned on occasion as a joke or feigned threat at times in the house. The device was traditionally used to punish sailors in the British Royal Navy. They were whipped on their bare backs; however, ship captains were only allowed to order up to 24 whips at a time.

Gregor's ex-wife is also British. He still has a piece of her lingerie that he keeps stashed in one of the drawers in the bedroom. It's red. One night I see Laura wearing it through the crack of the bedroom door. The strange thing about it is that Gregor's calling her by his ex-wife's name as if he's forgotten that she's his new wife. Apparently, one isn't enough for Gregor.

* * * * *

Toys may be the hallmark of BDSM to the vanilla world, which envisions whips and chains when they think of us, but to us, the hallmarks are consent and safety. Toys can indeed be a lot of fun, but it's also important to learn how to use them safely. We've all heard those horror stories about sex games gone wrong, but there's also the issue of sanitization that can get overlooked. And remember, just because someone has state-of-the-art fetish equipment doesn't mean that they know anything about safety. They may simply be what we in Los Angeles refer to as a "poser."

The sanitization issue that comes with toys has to do with fluid bonding. This practice ensures that all toys which come into contact with a person's bodily fluids are reserved for the exclusive use of that person and only that person. This includes dildos, butt plugs, and vibrators. Of course, they still need to be cleaned, but here's a word of caution about antibacterial sex toy cleaners: they often contain harsh disinfectants like benzalkonium chlorides (BAC or BKC) associated with significant vaginal irritancy. They're also very effective at killing lactobacillus, one of the essential kinds of healthy vaginal bacteria. Therefore, you might want to consider just using some warm water and soap for the task.

The following is a list of some BDSM toys, but please keep in mind that it is by no means a comprehensive one:

Blindfolds - Blindfolds are used during sensory deprivation. They can significantly heighten a person's physiological and psychological responses to other stimuli. By introducing an element of the unknown, a blindfold can add an air of excitement. It can also be used to create the impression of things occurring even when they're not.

Gags - Ball gags consist of a small ball made of rubber or silicone, which attaches to a securing strap. The true value lies in its psychological effect. It can create a sense of humiliation and helplessness. Another type of gag is a pony bit that's often used in BDSM pony play. It usually consists of a short narrow rod that is placed between the teeth. It also has straps attached at each end which can be secured around a person's head to hold it in place.

Whips - A common single-tail whip comes in three basic styles: bullwhip, stockwhip, and snakewhip. The bullwhip is probably one of the best known types of single-tail whip, but it's also one of the most difficult to learn how to use. A stockwhip has a long rigid handle that's connected to the lash by a leather swivel joint. A snakewhip doesn't have a rigid handle to be coiled up like a snake. The longer the whip, the less accurate the strike, which could cover the body's unintended areas. You should also keep in mind that a whip can cut like a knife when used too aggressively.

Crops - Crops, such as riding crops or horsewhips, usually consist of a long and slender flexible shaft, thicker at one end to form a handle and thinner at the other end to form a tongue or "keeper" of leather, cord, or neoprene. The flexible shaft adds speed and leverage to the strike, while the keeper is designed to come into contact with the target easily. Crops are often used to deliver stinging strikes against sensitive areas of the body, such as nipples or genitals. Still, they can be used practically anywhere else on the body as well.

Floggers - A flogger usually consists of a short-handled whip with multiple strips of leather or tails. It may also be referred to as a cat o' nine tails or lash. You'll want to choose your flogger based on the amount of impact you want to deliver, which can range from "slappy" to "stinging" however, floggers usually are not very pain-inflicting.

Canes - Canes are pretty simple in design and usually run about 2 feet in length. They may have a straight or curved handle and may or may not have a tassel at the end, which allows for different striking styles. Like the paddle, they're usually made of wood but can also consist of bamboo or plastic. The proper strike requires a skilled user, as cane strikes will almost always sting, but the degree of pain will be controlled through the proper technique. Some use a mix of strokes that sting and painless taps for maximum pleasure.

Paddles - A paddle usually consists of a short plank of wood, which has both a handle and a wide end that forms the blade, but it could also be made of bamboo, plastic, or metal. When using a paddle, make sure only to strike the muscled or fatty tissues of the body, such as the buttocks or thighs. You should also make sure you're using the paddle's flat side, taking care that the blade is parallel to the surface of the skin. This ensures that the force of the strike is evenly distributed across the breadth of the paddle blade. If there's even the slightest angle during the strike, it could be much more painful and may even cause severe damage.

Bondage Gear - The idea behind bondage gear is restricting a person's mobility, but never to the point of numbness, poor circulation, cutting, or pinching. This is why you should never leave the person alone once they've been bound. The most common use is for the restraint of the person's arms and legs, but it can also restrain the neck, head, torso, feet, hands, and genitalia. Some of the most common types of bondage gear are wrist and ankle cuffs, thumb cuffs, handcuffs, thigh cuffs, shackles, and zip ties for hog tying. The use of wrist and ankle cuffs can sometimes force the person's body into a position that causes postural asphyxiation or difficulty breathing.

Bondage Tape - Bondage tape is a relatively new toy on the scene. This revolutionary type of polymer tape sticks only to itself, but not to hair or skin. It can be used to gag, bind, blindfold, or completely mummify a person if so desired. Bondage tape is also reusable if you're up to rerolling it. Just make sure not to apply it so tightly that it restricts blood circulation.

Sleeves - A sleeve usually consists of a long tube made out of soft leather or canvas with buckles or straps and is sewn closed at one end. It's designed for the immobilization of one or both arms, typically behind the person's back. Sleeves are usually attached with buckles, straps, or O-rings. Sleeves immobilize the arms in a much more effective way than wrist cuffs. You should keep in mind that raising the attached arms too high behind the back or placing too much stress on them can cause a dislocation.

Straps, Chains & Ropes - Apparatuses like straps can be used to attach cuffs, sleeves, and collars to bedposts, etc. Just make sure the straps aren't ratcheted down too tightly. Chain is suitable for supporting heavy loads, but it's also heavy to use and can pinch the skin. Rope isn't just used in Japanese rope bondage; it's also a connector. You'll find that braided or nylon rope works best.

Harnesses - A harness is worn around the torso, to which you attach other things, such as dildos, chastity belts, or cock and ball torture devices. They can also be used with BDSM equipment, such as fetish furniture, hoists, swings, or other devices. They're used to attach your body to something else.

Spreader Bars - Spreader bars are designed for one purpose only: to keep a person's legs spread wide apart to provide easy access to their genitals. The device consists of a metal bar with rings at each end, to which ankle or wrist cuffs can be attached. Once again, you'll want to make sure to watch out for numbness and lack of blood circulation.

Racks - Racks have been around for over two thousand years. They were used for torture and perhaps even execution. The traditional rack usually resembled a wooden table with cylinders or ratcheting rollers at each end. Cables, ropes, or chains were attached to the ratcheting rollers, which were, in turn, attached to ankle or wrist cuffs. Ratcheting of the rollers put agonizing tension on the legs and arms, often until the point of severing body parts. Today's racks also stretch a person out by their wrists and ankles, but only to immobilize her while other things are being done to her.

Cages - Cages are sometimes used as punishment, but they can also be used as a holding cell. For example, there may come a time when a Dominant needs a few moments to think because he hasn't fully prepared for a scene. So, in the cage you go. And how big is your cage? Well, cages can be built to conform to the human body's size, so they restrict movement, they can be constructed in the shape of a box, and they can even be hoisted in the air. An entire room can even be transformed into a giant cage by simply installing a jail cell door with bars.

If you're worried about small prying eyes in the house, you might want to consider keeping your BDSM toys tucked away in the base of a bed frame that's built for such a purpose. They're even large enough to hide a person, though I wouldn't suggest doing so for an extended period.

‿ Chapter 14 ‿

Taskmaster II
(The Sadist Boss)

My Sadist Boss — Asa was a stuntman from the early days of Hollywood. He found cars that were good for the kind of stunts directors wanted in films. If you wanted an army truck that would blow up on the set, Asa would wire a bomb and weld a strapping device to secure it inside the truck. If you wanted a car to look like it had been underwater for a year, Asa would apply a seaweed treatment to the outside of the vehicle to make it appear as if the car had become part of the underwater landscape.

Asa was a talented genius with a permanent sneer and a black heart. Half the time, his mind raced with new ways to perform stunts. The other half the time, it raced with new ways to torment me, his assistant. One way was to monitor the number of bathroom breaks he saw me take on the 9-screen camera display on the warehouse wall. "Stop drinking so much water," he'd order me in the middle of 113-degree summer heat. "You're spending too much time in the bathroom and not enough time working." Another way he tormented me was to fill my lunch break with car wash runs, so there wouldn't be any time left for me to eat. Meanwhile, he had me pick up his lunch from the local diner whenever he got hungry.

I wasn't the only one who suffered Asa's wrath. Bank tellers had to listen to the same rant from him every week. "Why do you need to see my I.D.? Do you know who I AM?" he'd shout in a voice loud enough for everyone in the bank to hear. "Go get your supervisor! I'll have you fired!"

School employees at his son's school were bullied in the same way. If the bus driver was even ten minutes late returning from his son's high school soccer game, Asa would give him an ultimatum. "If you're ten minutes late one more time, I'll pull my son off this team!" he'd threaten as if the bus driver could control the length of the kids' soccer game.

Then there was the temperature setting of the window air conditioning unit in my office. The first thing Asa did each morning was crank it up to high, so it would blow directly onto me and into his office. No matter how heavy a coat I put on, my face would freeze and my hands would stiffen as I typed on the computer keyboard. Meanwhile, the sun would beat down on the four hundred cars in the lot outside until the dashboards cracked and the paint peeled. My last day of work came when Asa's son had finally had enough of his torment and threatened to bring a gas can and set the warehouse on fire.

* * * * *

So what are the signs of a sadist boss? Although you won't really know a person until you spend some time with them, you can certainly take some precautionary steps. This is where the Internet can be your ally. Do some searches for reviews of the establishment on websites such as Glassdoor. This is a site where current and former employees anonymously review companies, which can be very insightful.

For example, is there a review of your prospective boss that says he treats people more like inmates than employees? Has he denied his employees breaks? Maternity leave? Sick pay?

Also, ask about the cameras at the establishment and make sure to take a look around during the interview. Do you see any? If so, are they pointed toward the door, the parking lot, or your new desk? Are they small dome cameras in the corners of the room, or do they have large display screens on the wall for constant viewing? Make sure to also take a bathroom break during the interview and have a look around. Has a shower been installed in the bathroom so there's little need for the employees to ever leave and go home? Will you be expected to clean the bathroom and office floors along with your secretarial duties, perhaps on your hands and knees?

You might also want to ask how long the last employee worked for your prospective boss, as well as the employees before them. Does he have anything nice to say about them, or does he trash them to the point of resorting to profanity? And how does he feel about dirty jokes at the office? You may not want to ask him this, but pay attention if he tells you one during your interview. If so, this might be behavior that occurs daily, with each joke getting dirtier and dirtier until you're the butt of the joke.

Another prudent step would be to visit the neighboring businesses and get a feel for their opinion of your prospective boss. After all, you've probably included your references on your resume, so why not check out his? Most people don't make enemies everywhere they go, but you'll find that a sadist has a way of rubbing people the wrong way to the point that they won't be able to hold back their feelings about him when asked.

You'll also want to be aware of boundaries when you're considering working for someone new. For example, does your prospective boss stand too close to you when he's showing you around the new business? Does he ask you questions about your personal situation, such as your love life and whether you have a significant other? Will you be asked to travel? If so, will you get your own hotel room or will you be expected to be his "work wife?"

You may not think that sadists are very common in society, and perhaps they're not, but they're out there. It's been speculated that one in every 25 people is a sociopath, and while not every sadist is a sociopath, and not every sociopath is a sadist, do you really want to risk spending eight or more hours per day with one that's both? Do your homework. Check online and ask around before going to work for someone you don't know. After all, you wouldn't go on a date with someone without first taking some precautions, would you? Either venture could lead to a long-term relationship, so any time spent researching will be time well spent.

∞ Chapter 15 ∞

Taskmaster III
(The Dominant Boss)

My Dominant Boss — Gino was an aloof film producer from the early days of Hollywood. He started as a screenwriter and went on to produce R-rated films. If you were looking for sex to drip from the screen, Gino was your guy. If you wanted a nautical scene, Gino would shoot a woman naked and screaming underwater. If you wanted a cliff scene, Gino would shoot an actress bound and hanging from a knotted rope. I was Gino's production assistant.

Gino was a talented filmmaker with a ruthless eye for insubordination. The slightest perceived infraction by his employees sent him off on a stern rant that left them cowering. Outside vendors would offer to find Gino's employees another job so they wouldn't have to suffer his wrath another day. "You need to get away from him," they'd say. "It's not a healthy environment." Many of Gino's employees came and went after he'd ruined one too many of their days, but those who stayed were there for decades.

First, there was the temperature of the air in Gino's loft studio. It had gotten down to the fifties one day when I finally looked up at the ceiling and saw the exposed rafters. The studio had been so professionally built out that I hadn't even noticed that there was no insulation. There was also no way to heat the coffee I'd brought for warmth or refrigerate any of the food I'd brought for lunch. The microwave in the kitchen was out of the question since my food might smell up the main house. And when I refilled my water bottle, it was from the bathroom sink.

When I worked for Gino, he'd often send me to pick up the film that had been delivered to post-production, but I soon began to realize it was like a game I couldn't win. If I left the film on the kitchen table, I'd get a text message from him saying that I should've let him know it was there. So the next time, I'd sent him a text and let him know I'd left the film on the table. But then I'd receive a text from him saying, "Thank you for letting me know, but I would've seen it when I went to the kitchen without you texting me."

Another day, I found myself in yet another uncomfortable situation involving the removal of my top. Gino had hired an actress for a film who had breasts that were an inadequate size. It was a sci-fi film, and he wanted them to really "pop" beneath the breast-plates, which were supposed to look like metal leaves holding the breasts. The actress was willing to have implants inserted to get the part; her only concern was that her new breasts felt real. "Deanna, yours are silicone, right? Take off your top and let her feel them," he ordered, turning around. I reluctantly did as instructed and soon felt the hands of a strange woman squeezing my breasts.

* * * * *

There are good Dominants, and there are bad Dominants out there. So, how do you spot a bad one before it's too late? Once again, you can check out some reviews on websites such as Glassdoor and ask around. Perhaps the bad Dominant won't go so far as to have cameras pointed at your desk or the bathroom door, but he'll still cause you a lot of pain. His games may be more about verbal abuse and unwanted devaluation than a violation of boundaries and physical risk. Therefore, you'll want to pay close attention to the tone he uses during your interview. Contradicting himself will be another red flag.

A good Dominant boss will mentor you and bring out the best in you, just as you might find in an internship situation. He'll also be consistent with his discipline and the doling out of rewards and punishment. He might use some mind games, but there should be some resolution and reassurance afterward. I, however, had only submitted to being Gino's employee; therefore, mind games had never been negotiated, much less aftercare. Gino and I had also never negotiated public humiliation or devaluation. Do your research before working for someone because you never know what you're going to get.

✌ Chapter 16 ✃

Domestic Service

My Dominant — After my first dinner with Zane, we walk out to the Strand, and he takes me by surprise by placing his large hand on my throat and kissing me passionately. What's he doing holding my throat like this? I wonder, but it's turning me on. He has full lips that hold each kiss for several moments, savoring them as we stand together in the night air. I've never done this with anyone before. Before I know it, he's directing me over to his car. "Get in for a minute," he orders.

I do as he says and am barely able to pull the door closed before he starts up once again with the kisses. The privacy of the car's interior shields us from onlookers and allows Zane to tug at me and reel me in. Thankfully he doesn't try to feel inside my shirt, for I'm nowhere near ready for that. But I know it's coming.

I text Zane when I get home just like he's asked and assure him I'm safe. But am I? Why do I freeze up at the thought of becoming more intimate with him? I can't imagine him getting past my boundaries and peeling off my clothes. I already feel so exposed with them on when he touches me. Maybe I need some more therapy for my PTSD. No, there's no time for that. My life is passing me by, and I need to buck up and be a woman. Somehow I'm going to get past my intimacy issues.

"I have a fantasy about you against my wall. Would you like to hear about it?" Zane asks in his text back to me.

"What?" I reluctantly reply.

"I pull your arms up over your head and hold them there," he continues.

I don't respond.

"And then I kiss you. That's it," he concludes, sensing my hesitation.

I head into the bathroom, run some water in the tub, and light some candles. Oh, how I love my bath time. I can shut out the world and lose myself in the bubbles. No phone, no interruptions, no obligations. Just me and the white steam with my head thrown back against the bathroom wall. I wonder if Zane has a tub or just a shower at his house. Soon he'll find out what a prude I am, I think, and maybe lose interest in me. I'm determined not to let that happen, but he's definitely going to have to be patient. Once the drawbridge finally lowers, the castle will be open, and there'll be no turning back for this Cinderella.

* * * * *

My first memory of domestic service to a boy my own age dates back to when I was sixteen. It was summertime and a bunch of us from the neighborhood had gone tubing at our friend's lake house. I remember one of the girls coming to me in the bedroom and confiding that she'd overheard my boyfriend tell his friends to watch while he ordered me to bring him a bowl of chili. "Don't do it," she warned. "He's bragging to all his friends that you're his slave."

"But I want to do it," I told her. So I did, while all his friends watched in amazement as I did exactly what he'd told me to do.

Not all D/s relationships include domestic service. Some keep their power exchange confined to the bedroom, which is fine as long as that's what both partners want. Having a power exchange in the bedroom but a power struggle outside the bedroom isn't going to work, so this should be negotiated upfront.

As I've said before, this book is written from the perspective of a female sub in service to a male Dominant, and males and females are two very different biological creatures. Females produce and secrete two main hormones—estrogen and progesterone. Estrogen includes the increased tendency for nurturing and maternal behavior, and progesterone is the hormone that prepares for and maintains pregnancy. Testosterone is the primary sex hormone found in men. It fuels both competition and protectiveness. So you can see that these make for two very opposing roles. This doesn't mean that a female is not capable of competing in a man's world. That's not what I'm saying at all; I'm merely saying that this is not her primary biological function. That being said, if a male goes out into the world, competes with others, and brings home a larger share of the bacon, perhaps the female may wish to serve him in some comparable way. Obviously this isn't always the case, but it's an example of restoring the balance between the two roles. Therefore, it sheds light on the motivation behind some domestic service.

One of the ways you can begin your domestic service is with a frilly apron. You can find one online and buy it yourself or send the link to your Dominant and ask him to purchase it for you. You might also ask him to tie the apron on you the first time. That way you'll be sure to remember the experience.

You can also wear French maid outfits while you're cooking and cleaning, and a plastic carryall for cleaning supplies can be a handy accessory. These are both optional, of course, and the outfits will be impractical during the winter when it's cold. They will, however, be greatly appreciated by your Dominant, who will reserve the right to interrupt your service to him at any time for BDSM sex. Perhaps he'll lay you out on top of the pile of unfolded laundry. If so, make sure not to complain about the fact that the clothes may get wrinkled. You can also expect him to ask you this question: "Why are you here?" to which you should answer: "To serve and service you, Sir."

The lingerie needn't stop with the French maid outfit, either. You might want to spend some time browsing the Internet to find your favorite slutty lingerie shop. Remember, the lingerie needn't be quality, nor should it be, as your Dominant reserves the right to rip your outfit off you at any time. This is why it pays to spend the time searching for a shop that provides deep discounts and shallow quality. You may not be in that $7 outfit for very long, so it's better not to have spent a fortune on it.

Purchasing a service notebook is also optional, but it may be helpful when providing domestic service for an extremely particular Dominant. The first page, which may read: Service Notebook for _____ in service to _____, may be torn out to maintain privacy if you like. So may any pages that don't apply to your particular relationship or household. You might want to spend some time browsing online to find just the right service notebook that suits your needs. Perhaps you want a spiral notebook for convenience or one with a hardcover that you can have embossed.

Your service notebook helps you keep track of your Dominant's information and preferences. Unless you have a photographic memory, you'll find one helpful. I, myself, find it helpful to keep track of certain wines that my Dominant likes with certain foods. I also purchased a book on wine pairing after he declared it my job to select the wine to go with the food each evening. It's also my job to ensure that the wine has been placed in the fridge (or freezer temporarily) to ensure it's served at the right temperature. If you find that your Dominant drinks wine but you are not exactly a connoisseur, you might find it helpful to study a book on wine pairings and record suggested pairings in your service notebook. For example, perhaps a sparkling Fume Blanc is said to pair well with Indian food, but you find that your Dominant prefers a flinty Chardonnay after trying it out. You may also find it helpful to list both a suggested wine and preferred wine. That way you'll have options should you run out of one kind.

These are some of the sections that you will find in most service notebooks: Home, Tasks, Housework, Food, Shopping, People, Hobbies & Interests, Entertaining, Travel, Vehicles, Medical Information, Children, and Recordkeeping & Finances. The shopping list should be updated each time an item is almost empty, and oft-used items should have backups. I've taken gourmet cooking classes and highly recommend them. You may also want to educate yourself about wine storing procedures and devices.

♋ Chapter 17 ♋

Sexting

"So, how was the second date?" my friend, Barry, asks me about Deanna.

I sigh a frustrated sigh. "I don't know, she's so... cold. I don't know if she's ever going to warm up," I tell him.

"A frigid one, huh? That's a new one for you," Barry cracks. He knows how I like my women—willing.

"You going to see her again?"

"Yeah, I am, but next time I'm going to make her come back to my place," I state.

"Going to drag her back to the cave, huh? Well, let me know how it goes."

"I will," I promise.

Deanna's not the kind of woman I usually go for, that's for sure. I like them to be a little more demonstrative, a little more affectionate. There's something about her, though, but I can tell that phone sex isn't an option, which is something I like to do on occasion. A few getting to know them texts, a few jokes, and then turn on Skype. There you can check out things like the nipples. Oh, how I love them long—long enough to tie them together. The longer the better.

One woman even challenged me in the past. She wanted to see if I could make her come on-screen. I had to take her up on that one. First I had her unbutton her blouse, then show me her bra. Then I had her take one of her breasts out. Her nipple had been a decent size, not extra long, but functional. I told her to put it in her mouth, then I had her put one hand down her panties and rub on her clit while I watched from the screen. I had my hand on my cock as well, rubbing it as I told her what a good job she was doing. She made my cock extra hard and I pulled on it until my seed shot up my stomach and came into her view. That made her happy; she came and I won the bet. Then I made her stand up and show herself to me.

My last relationship had been intense and short-lived. Very intense. Bailey had been bipolar and in need of a lot of discipline. At only five feet tall, I'd been able to pin her against my wall, which had left her feet dangling beneath her. She'd liked it rough—rougher than even I was used to—but I was able to compartmentalize my usual behaviors and accommodate her. The problems had all been outside the bedroom. I had wanted control both inside and out, but she didn't see herself as a full-time submissive. In the end, she'd hit me in the arm with her purse and run out of the restaurant alone.

I'm used to having things my way and don't tolerate disobedience in a woman, which has often led to problems. Lately I've decided that the best thing to do is just be clear about this in the beginning. If a woman wants to walk after that, so be it, because eventually she will. My rules are strict and I'm very particular about the way I like things: my house, my food, and especially my sex. Sometimes I will entertain suggestions, but only if I happen to be in the mood. Outside of that, I am both the director and the producer.

* * * * *

Sexual arousal is a vital element of a sub's job in the world of BDSM. Most women are aware that men have a higher sex drive than them but the degree to which this is true often escapes them. The testosterone production in men may be as high as 20 times the levels in women, which can shed a whole new light on the subject. Males generally think about sex twice as often as females, which can lead to their mind wandering when they encounter one. They may ponder thoughts about a woman's vagina, such as: Is it active? Is it moist? Is it swollen? Many of us have heard of a man staring at a woman's breasts while she's talking to him rather than listening to what she has to say. We've also likely heard the expression "he's undressing her with his eyes." Testosterone will be the guilty party in each of these incidents.

A sub should be aware that her Dom may be masturbating anywhere between two and ten times per day. He's likely pleasuring himself at least once in the morning upon awakening and once at night before he goes to sleep. Regular masturbation not only releases built-up sexual tension but also relieves stress and improves sleep. Therefore a sub should realize her duties are not confined to the physical act of sex with her Dom. There may also be times when he's traveling or simply sleeping in a different location should he reside alone. This is when sexting can come into play.

Initiation of an erection occurs generally through stimulation of nerves but this doesn't mean it's solely due to the result of touch. Sexual thoughts or visual stimulation can result in an erection as well. This is where you, the sub, could come in. You could send an erotic photo of yourself in sexy red lingerie to your Dom, or better yet, send an entire photoshoot of you in various stages of removal of the pieces. For example, the second photo could show you without the stockings, the third photo could show you without the bra, etc. A striptease video could be an alternative option.

Then we have point of view (POV) photos. These little gems give the impression of actually being in the moment when it's not physically possible to do so. For example, you could snap a photo from the erotic point of view of the removal of your top to the shake of your booty. You could even tease your Dom with a close-up photo of your nipples beneath a sheer blouse. The open vagina POV will go a long way as well. You could start by giving your Dom a peek of your "pink" by sliding over a G-string or pair of lace panties with your finger. You could also switch up the color or mix and match the panties with a neon mesh top. Next, you could remove the panties and spread your vaginal lips open with your fingers or spread open your legs.

If you really want to crank up the heat, you could film a masturbation video or "solo" where you could cum on screen for your Dom and maybe even squirt (this is the "money shot"). You could also break out the BDSM gear and put on your collar or spank yourself with a paddle. Add in a dildo, vibrator, or some of the toys from the toy chapter for some extra spice. You could even go for different colors or different features to mix it up. If you're daring enough to try interactive play, there are remote control vibrators that you and your Dom can use via the computer.

If you care to go the extra mile and pull back the camera, there's the arching "backshot" photo. For this shot, you raise your ass in the air and turn back to look at the camera. You could also pull on a pair of youthful knee socks and sit on the kitchen counter with your legs open or snap a photo of yourself in spandex after a sweaty workout. The possibilities are endless.

You can see that with a little effort, your Dom can remain captivated by you even when you're not around. Remember, a smartphone can go a long way. If you're self-conscious about your figure, you can accentuate your better features and touch up the photos with a photo editing app. Professional models do this all the time and so can you.

Keep in mind, however, that photos and videos are only part of a whole when it comes to the world of BDSM. Remember the dirty talk you and Dom use during power exchange? This is where video chats or sexting could come in. The two of you could sext back and forth together, you could give your Dom a video with jerk-off instructions (JOI), or you could have a one-sided sexting session where you create a scene. The following is an example of the latter.

May I please please suck your cock, Sir?

And pull on the head nice and slowww?

Am I to be allowed pleasure, Sir?

Or is the pleasure all for you?

I am but a lowly submissive.

I'm your property and I'm here to serve and service you.

Shall I sit on your face, Sir, or turn around?

Will you be putting it in my ass, Sir?

Will you please bind my wrists to the bed rail and I'll lie back on the bed, Sir?

I'm spreading my beautiful slutty legs wide for you, Sir…

(Insert sexy photo or video)

Ohhhhhh……. you're shoving your cock inside me, Sir……

It feels SOOOO good………

Mmmm……… ohhhhhhhhhhhh………..

Ohhhhhhhh...... OHHHHHHHHHHHH...

Thank you, Sir... my body is all for you...

It feels SOO fucking good......

I need to cum SOO bad...

I live to service you, Sir...... it's my only job......

Ohhhh! I'm cumming! I'm cumming SOOO fucking hard!

Mmmm....... will you be cumming inside me, Sir?

I feel your throbbing cock, Sir...

My pussy is vibrating around it... can you feel me, Sir?
I'm gripping your cock...

I need your cock SOOO much, Sir......

Mmmm......... ohhhhhhhhhhhh...........

Ohhhhhhhh...... OHHHHHHHHHHHH....................

Ohhhh! I'm cumming!

(Insert sexy photo or video)

You spoil me with your huge cock, Sir......

I will take it as you shove it down my throat, Sir...

Because it's my job to service you whenever you command...

I'm getting railed SOOOO HARD right now, Sir...

And I need it SOOO BAD because I'm such a fucking slut...

I can't even stand it sometimes, Sir...

Mmmmmmmm....... I feel your cock sliding in and out of me, Sir......

It makes me SOOO happy to be your little cumdumpster……

Does my pussy please you, Sir?

Am I worthy of your cum?

Please, Sir… please fill me up like the whore I am…

Thank you for allowing me to service you, Sir…

You can sext with your Dom as you go or create scripts in advance to have them ready at a moment's notice. It's a good rule of thumb to rotate them so that you're not using the same one each time. As long as you're having fun with it your Dom will be sure to have fun with it too. And if security's an issue for either of you, there are private photo apps you can use to keep your photos and videos hidden. Therefore there should be nothing to stop you from keeping your Dom aroused like a good submissive.

❦ Chapter 18 ⛥

Finding the Right Dominant

"Come with me," Zane orders. "I'm going to take you to my wall."

I rise from Zane's sofa and feel a tinge of excitement yet acceptance about whatever he has in mind for me. The amount of chemistry between us is astounding. We're in sync with one another. I take his hand and follow him into the hallway, where he leaves me for a moment. "Wait here. I'll be right back," he says. Soon he returns from the bedroom with a soft blindfold and necktie. "I'm going to put this blindfold on you and bind your wrists with this, but not too tightly," he explains so as not to frighten me.

I suddenly trust him completely and feel enveloped by a sense of calm. Zane slips the blindfold over my eyes and the hallway becomes dark. Then I feel the softness of a silk necktie against my wrists as he proceeds to bind them loosely this first time. Up over my head they go as Zane firmly presses them against the cold wall above my head. His kisses on my lips are even firmer and more urgent in their delivery. He keeps me in the hallway for several minutes. One hand pins my wrists, and the other finds my breast and then my nipple. Zane pulls on it and pinches, sending a twinge of pain up to my brain, which causes a fog to disburse. Then he leads me into the bedroom.

I feel strong hands on my shoulders. They push me back onto the bed into a seated position. Suddenly I'm falling backward onto the soft comforter behind me. Then I feel my legs being spread apart like scissors in the air—something I've never allowed him to do before. I've finally given up control and surrendered to my Dominant. It's something he questioned me about later after unearthing my past. "Why didn't you give up control to me right away?" he wanted to know. I told him it was because once it was gone, it would be gone.

* * * * *

Have you perhaps been searching for a Dominant but either haven't found one or have found the wrong one? If so, you're not alone, but you may need to take inventory of yourself. Here are some points to think about:

- Do you walk gracefully? Tilting your pelvis inward allows your shoulders to pull back and your head to lift with confidence. Good posture is very important.

- Do you wear dresses?

- Do you only speak about yourself when conversing with someone, or do you show interest in them and their life?

- Are you articulate when you speak and write?

- Do you have good manners at the table, or do you speak with your mouth full?

- Are you a positive person, or do you allow yourself to stay in a negative vibration when problems arise?

- Are you judgmental of others or supportive of them?

- Are you a spontaneous person or rigid?
- Do you give up easily or work to sustain a relationship?
- Have you studied consciousness and achieved spiritual growth?

You might want to browse the self-help aisle at your local bookstore or self-help videos on YouTube to get into the vibration to attract the kind of Dominant you want. I spent two years doing this, and it has completely changed my life. Remember that Albert Einstein said, "The definition of insanity is doing the same thing over and over again and expecting different results." Have you run into the same types of problems in your relationships over and over again? If so, they may have even manifested themselves in your dreams. This is because your dreams are trying to tell you something. Do the work on yourself.

So, what kind of traits would you like in your Dominant? Here are some to think about:

- Positive Attitude
- Loyalty
- Devotion
- Empathy
- Insight
- Stability
- Curiosity

And let's not forget values. You'll want your Dominant's values to be in line with yours. Does he value family? Loyalty? Trust? Does he value what's new? Hip? Trendy? Try asking some indirect questions to get a better idea of what's important to him. For example, you might want to run a hypothetical ethical dilemma by him and see what choice he would make. People are defined by their choices.

Communication is critical for a relationship. Think of it as throwing a ball to someone. Really, you just want to make sure that they "get it," but it's also important that they throw it back to you. However, we all have our different "catching" and "throwing" styles. Is your Dominant analytical? If so, he may be more apt to be persuaded by reason and analogies. If he's emotional, he may be more likely to be persuaded by emotion.

During my previous marriage, I used to kiss my husband goodbye on my way out to the gym. This was my way of letting him know that I was leaving the house. Unfortunately, it was also right in the middle of his work morning. He used to get up early before the stock market opened and would be engrossed in analyzing stock prices. My kiss, I began to notice, would break his concentration and annoy him. Eventually, I stopped interrupting him in this way and started leaving notes for him on the kitchen counter instead.

Has your Dominant ever been married? If so, do he and his ex-wife still get along? Is there a restraining order in place? If so, has he violated it? Does he ever accuse you of being just like his ex? If so, he may be encountering the same types of problems in each of his relationships and may need to do some work on himself. Are you aware that there are therapists who specialize in BDSM relationships? The two of you may even want to consider visiting one together.

And what about your former marriage? Did you and your spouse outgrow each other? Did you communicate well? If not, have you learned how to communicate more effectively? Did one of you do all the growing while the other stood still or regressed? Did one do all the nurturing while the other took without giving back? Perhaps you didn't have a D/s relationship with your ex and weren't even aware that you wanted one. Maybe you wished he'd been able to take control of you, but he lacked control in his own life. If this is the case, it's possible that he lacked your respect. Trust and respect are vital elements when it comes to a relationship.

Has your Dominant managed people at work? If so, how's his management style? Is he firm and nurturing? Does he listen to his associates' concerns? You might want to listen in on a conference call that he's having with his staff if he happens to do some of his work from home and you're able to do so. If so, you'll learn a lot about the management style he'll undoubtedly use with you.

When I was twenty-eight, I met a man at a hotel bar in South Florida. He'd flown in from California on a business trip, but he worked from home. We'd spent the weekend in South Beach, and he'd told me within the first hour that he was going to marry me. I'd brushed off the comment and quickly forgotten about it. After growing up in South Florida, I'd heard every line imaginable from men while working at restaurants on the intercoastal. But, sure enough, he'd flown me to California three weeks later, and I'd moved in with him. Suddenly I found myself living the life of a mail-order bride. "May I go to the gym?" I'd asked him soon after I'd arrived.

"Of course," he'd answered, pleased that I'd asked permission of him in this way. That's how my married life began, but it wasn't submission, and it didn't last.

Two years before I met my current Dominant, I'd decided to put all of my focus on myself and my kids and didn't date. Instead, I did a lot of therapeutic writing, took classes at the local university, and watched hundreds of documentaries about self-improvement and consciousness. I also practiced the art of pushing all negative thoughts out of my mind. It's been said that once you get to a point where you stop looking back, you're ready to move forward. So that's just what I did;

I went out and found my Dominant and the type of D/s relationship that I wanted.

So what are you looking for in a relationship? Role play? Lifestyle BDSM? 24/7 BDSM? Have a vision, make a plan, and go after it. Design your own BDSM world with your Dominant before handing over control. Make it as colorful as you both want it to be, and then get in the saddle. Only then will you enjoy the ride.

ℬ Reader Bonus ℭ

A teaser of
Deanna Hankel's memoir

Trapped in the 70s: Behind A Sadist's Door

* * *

Chapter 1

House Rules

Gregor is from Liverpool, England. He arrived in the United States in the late 1960s and purchased a home in South Florida. His first marriage to a fellow Brit lasted a mere two years, then ended in divorce. The two no longer speak. Gregor has mutton chop sideburns, a charcoal-colored mustache, and dark tinted glasses with teardrop frames. It's now the 1970s and, like other competing males of the decade, Gregor likes to wear his shirt partially unbuttoned to reveal the hair on his tanned chest. He finishes off the look with a gold chain, which makes him look like someone who works in the porn industry.

Gregor pulls his white Camaro into the driveway of his house and crushes out his cigarette in the ashtray. He grabs his European man-purse from the red leather passenger seat. It contains, among other items, his membership card to a swinger's club. Gregor never parks his car in the garage; he prefers to keep that area dark and empty. He likes his house and gets smug satisfaction out of the fact that he lives right next door to the fire department. If they only knew what was going on in the house right next door. But they don't, and he plans to keep it that way.

Baine, Gregor's full-grown black Doberman Pinscher, is waiting for his Master behind the side gate just like he does every day. The dog bares his large fangs in a smile for Gregor and begins licking his arm. "That's right, I'm home, Boy. Are you ready for your Master to take you out for a walk?" Gregor asks his pet. He steps into the small garage and grabs Baine's leash from its hook on the wall. There's no need to turn on the light; he knows just where it is.

The house is solid. The two-bedroom home was built out of white concrete block and made for hurricane weather. The Florida room has been fashioned out of the screened-in patio. It's Gregor's pride and joy. It houses his black and white bar and two high-backed leather bar stools. Baine often curls up in one of the two matching black leather saucer chairs by the TV. The room's interior sliding glass doors have been pushed together toward the center so that one can step down onto the bright orange shag carpet of the Florida room on either side. Orange is a popular color in 1976. It offsets the avocado green carpet in the living room and the appliances in the kitchen. Many 1970s households use the same color scheme, but the similarities stop there. Gregor plays by his own rules.

For one, there's the nude sunbathing that Gregor enjoys on the folding chaise lounge chair in his backyard on the concrete deck. Occasionally it falls into shadow from the umbrella table, so he has to drag the chair out onto the grass.

Then he can resume basking in the Florida sun. Tall rubber tree plants wall the yard along with a few pink and yellow hibiscus flowers. No one can see into the yard from any of the sides of the fence. Not that Gregor would be the slightest bit embarrassed should they peek. He's quite proud of his all-over dark tan. Even his uncircumcised penis doesn't cause him any shame. British men only get the cut for religious or medical reasons, and he certainly isn't religious.

Gregor's only religion is nudism. It's something he's been practicing since the closest nudist camp, Sun Gardens, opened back in 1972. His ex-wife, Diana, hadn't shared his enthusiasm for nudism. Nor had she shared enthusiasm for his brand of S&M. After she'd left, Gregor had placed an ad in the local newspaper, the *Sun Sentinel*, that read:

**Sadist seeking masochist for bondage,
swinging, and more.**

Laura, a divorced single mother, had answered his ad.

Laura was from South Carolina, but she'd relocated to South Florida with her ex-husband for his work. He'd been into heavy domination, so the descent into S&M had hardly been a downward spiral. She'd worn glasses, bell-bottom jeans, and a shy smile for Gregor when they'd met. Malleable was the term that came to mind, like a beaten puppy in need of house training. House training in Gregor's house. She had a little blond daughter who seemed very demure as well. A pretty little thing. The two of them would make fine additions to Gregor's household, he decided.

* * * * *

"Out of the way, Baine. Let Laura and Deanna come inside," Gregor orders his dog. Baine blocks the front doorway and continues barking. It takes him a minute or two to finally calm down. "Deanna, put your stuff in the first bedroom on the left. That's your room now," Gregor announces in his British accent.

Laura heads back out to the moving truck for another box. The move takes several hours. The sun goes down before the truck is finally driven back to the rental store. When they all return, Gregor has an announcement for Laura. "This is my house and you will follow my rules. We are now a nudist family and will not wear clothes in the house." He goes on to explain that even on a rare winter day when it happens to be cold, permission is to be asked of him to wear clothes. And he may say no. "Do you understand?" he asks.

"Yes, Master," Laura dutifully replies.

"What are you?" Gregor asks next.

"I am your slave, Master."

"And why are you my slave?"

"Because I have given up all of my rights and property to you," Laura concedes.

"That's right. You have. Now go unpack your things," Gregor instructs. He watches Laura turn down the short hallway and head into the master bedroom. Then he slips into the kitchen and cracks some ice cubes into a glass.

Once he reaches the Florida room, Gregor slips behind the bar. He grabs a bottle of Boodles British Gin, pours a couple of shots over ice, then takes a good long swig. After that, he lights a cigarette and takes a very long drag.

Gregor does as he pleases. Always. He listens to the sound of the boxes being cut open in the bedrooms, takes another drag from his cigarette, and plots his next move.

References

Cunningham, Kacie. *Conquer Me*. Greenery Press, Inc., 2010.

Easton, Dossie, and Janet W. Hardy. *Radical Ecstasy: S/M Journeys in Transcendence (Mind Journeys Chapter)*. Greenery Press, 1879.

Huntsman, Skyeler. "The Extended History of BDSM." *Https://Historymsu.Wordpress.Com/*, 2017, https://historymsu.wordpress.com/2017/04/26/the-extended-history-of-bdsm/.

Larsen, Brooke. "BDSM Is Older Than You Think. Way Older." *Https://Www.Kinkly.Com/*, 2019, https://www.kinkly.com/bdsm-is-older-than-you-think-way-older/2/17777.

Makai, Michael. The BDSM Relationship Handbook. Michael Makai, 2013.

Rubel Ph.D., Robert J.. Master/Slave Relations. Nazca Plains Corporation, 2007.

Rubel Ph.D., Robert J.. Protocols Handbook for the Female Slave. Nazca Plains Corporation, 2007.

Sehayek, Marnie. "A Brief History of Japanese Rope Bondage." *Https://Www.Vice.Com/*, 2017, Sehayek, Marnie. Kinbaku-Japanese-Rope-Bondag. Https://Www.Vice.Com. 2017.

Swensen, Michele. "The Astonishing History of Journaling." *Https://Epica.Com/*, 2018, https://epica.com/blogs/epica-news/the-astonishing-history-of-journaling.

Technogeisha, Miko. "Sensual Mind Games & Giving Up Control – Humiliation in BDSM and Kink." *Https://Www.Lifeontheswingset.Com/*, 2012, https://www.lifeontheswingset.com/11279/sensual-mind-games-and-giving-up-control-humiliation-in-bdsm-and-kink/.

Thesexblogger, Robyn. "What Is Flogging? Ancient Punishment Vs Modern Kink." *Https://Www.Lovense.Com/*, 2020, https://www.lovense.com/bdsm-blog/what-is-flogging.

Thorne, Morgan. "Ask – Verbal Humiliation Ideas." *Http://Msmorganthorne.Com/*, 2018, http://msmorganthorne.com/ask-verbal-humiliation-ideas/.